Traditional Chinese
Brews & Remedies

Published by
Landmark Books Pte Ltd
5001 Beach Road
#02-73/74
Singapore 199588

Landmark Books is an imprint of Landmark Books Pte Ltd

ISBN 978-981-4189-26-2

Printed in Singapore

Traditional Chinese Brews & Remedies

Ng Siong Mui

·LANDM△RK·BOOKS·

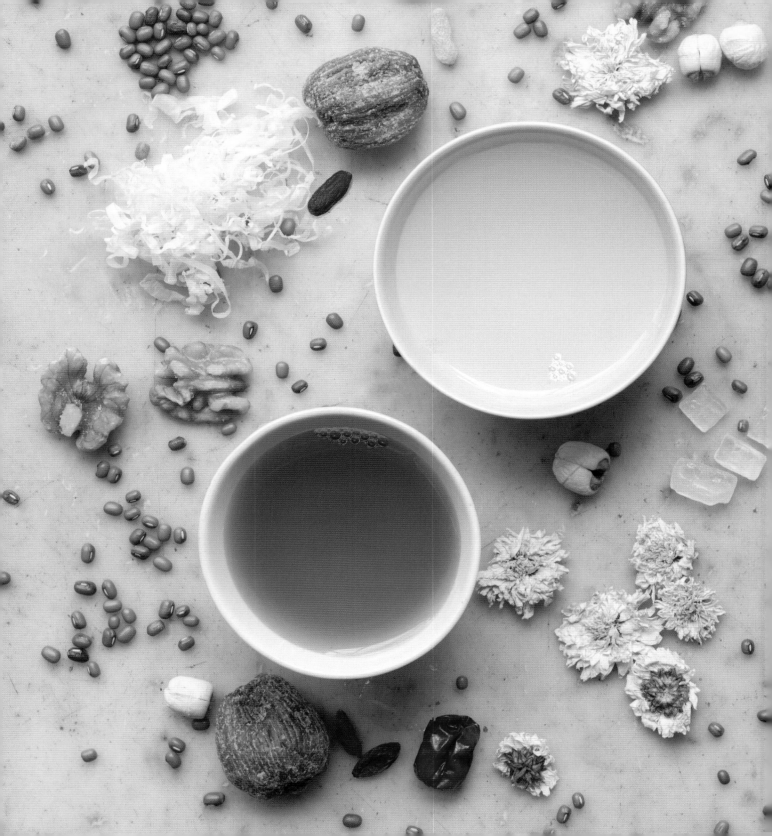

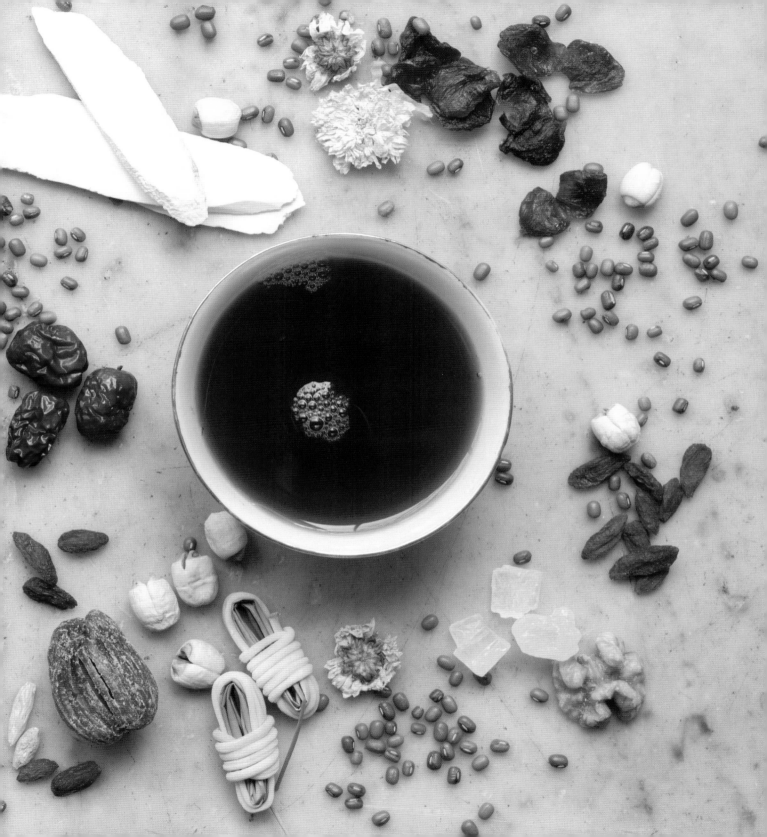

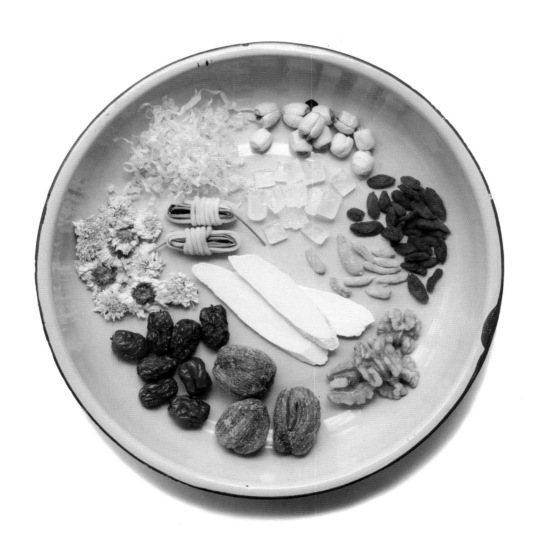

PREFACE

Since I was a child, I have been fascinated by the food served to me. Grandmother and Mother were the cooks of our family while Father was the chef in his own restaurant. So, from a tender age, my siblings and I have enjoyed healthy home-cooking as well as delectable banquet fare.

At the age of four, I began to follow my father on his routine trips to the market in Chinatown. We rode on a trishaw, and a regular stop was to buy Chinese herbal ingredients and have a long chitchat with his best friend, Doctor Tong Wah Tat. Doctor Tong was a qualified physician from China and was the in-house doctor of Kung Soon Loong Herbal Shop. Through Father's influence, I began to look up to Doctor Tong as my mentor. I was fascinated by his profession. He was the first to tell me about the yin and yang characteristics in people. I told myself then that I wanted to be like him, telling others, "You are yang and heaty, you are yin and cooling."

In secondary school, I majored in Home Economics and my love for cookery deepened. Later, I married a herbalist. From 1973, through my contact with herbalists and food therapists in China, I began researching the properties of different herbs and ingredients, analysing them according to Chinese food concepts. It is a subject based on food eaten to please the palate, to demonstrate culinary skills, and for health.

I have covered different aspects of healthy Chinese food in my other books: *Secrets of Chinese Nutrition*, *The Chinese Pregnancy and Confinement Cookbook*, *Nutritious Chinese Food for Infants, Children and Youth*, and *The Chinese Health, Beauty and Rejuvenation Cookbook*.

Here, I would like to share with you some of my family's food remedies which we have used for generations. They have proven useful to my household and will be useful to you too, even though you do not need them every day.

If you are Chinese, I am sure that you would have encountered a few of these remedies at home. You might have been given a bowlful of soup or brew without any explanation other than "drink this, it is good for you." These remedies are not old wives' tales. From time immemorial, food concepts have been a unique part of Chinese culture and science through empirical practice. Through my research, I have found that Chinese scholars and pharmacologists have recorded the reasons for eating various foods, and there is sound basis for even the simplest home brew.

The only strange thing is that the recipes for these remedies are seldom found in books. Rather, they were passed down orally from generation to generation. Through this book, I hope to preserve these recipes and make them accessible to anyone who is interested in maintaining good health the natural, Chinese way.

Ng Siong Mui

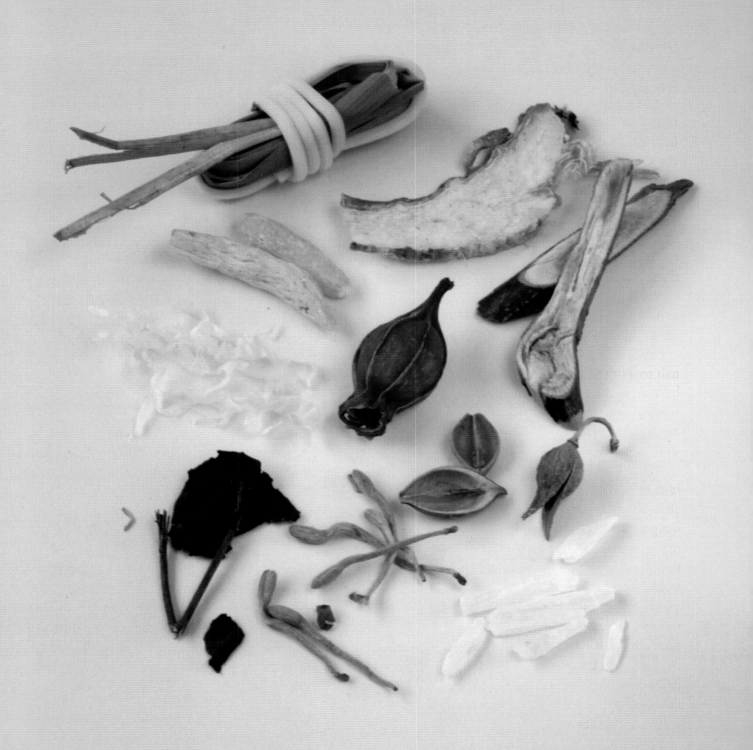

INTRODUCTION

In the agrarian society of old China, most people could not afford to stay in the sickbed for long. In fact, they literally could not afford to be ill. As the Chinese saying goes: "hands stop, mouth stops." In other words, when one is sick, there would be no work, hence there would be no income to buy food. It was also difficult for the largely farming communities to reach physicians, and one was only summoned when someone was very ill. Even in the days when I was growing up in Chinatown in Singapore, I saw people living in such poverty that they could not afford to consult a doctor. But like the farmers of old, they survived.

So, what happened when people felt that they were falling ill, or when they were already sick? They relied on traditional Chinese brews and remedies.

My family was fortunate to have been able to call on a doctor when we had to, but the elders still gave us food remedies. In fact, there seemed to be a brew or tea for the slightest discomfort. Whenever someone fell ill or was starting to feel unwell, the elder ladies in the neighbourhood would inevitably gather and exchange recipes for remedies. As children, my siblings and I were fascinated with some of the remedies that were applied.

Neighbours and friends would come by to borrow Father's silver belt buckle to boil in hot water in order to make a brew. We were told that after an accident or shock, when young children became fretful in their sleep or cried continuously as a result, even developing a fever, a brew made with a silver object, such as Father's belt buckle, may help to calm them down (定惊). The cleaned buckle would then be returned together with a red packet of cash as a token of thanks.

One of my strongest childhood memories was of Grandmother testing to see if someone had *mo tan* toxins. *Mo tan* (毛丹) literally means hair-pore toxins. It is a condition where the body heat of a very heaty person is completely locked in his body system. Toxins cannot leave the body and just circulate continuously. The result is high fever, influenza with body fatigue, and aches for many days.

Grandmother would make a dough with a cup of sieved glutinous rice flour and the white of an egg, then use it to rub the chest and back of the person for two minutes. Then she would break open the dough. There would be very fine golden 'hairs' in it if the toxins were present.

To draw out the toxins, Grandmother would get a kilogram of chicken feathers from the market. She would wash the feathers clean and put them in a pail half-filled with boiling water. After cooling it for five minutes, she would take handfuls of the hot, wet feathers and rub them briskly on the person, starting from the face, down the body to the toes, including all the limbs and especially the joints. After ensuring there are no feathers stuck to the body, she would take a meter of black cloth and use short, brisk downward strokes to dry the body thoroughly. It is still a mystery to me, but golden 'threads' and tiny silver 'scales'– the toxins drawn out from the body's open pores, she said – would appear on the black cloth.

Boiling silver belt buckles? Hair-pore toxins? These stories will likely sound like nonsensical fairy tales to some of you. Tests and scientific evidence may not yet be available to show how these remedies work, but they already have more modern standing than we might previously have imagined. Silver has been found to be a powerful disinfectant with antiseptic properties and is now commonly employed in nanotechnology for household products as well as external wound dressings in hospitals. As for the removal of hair-pore toxins, our skin is the largest human organ with a built-in function for the excretion of body waste through sweating. It makes sense then, that when toxins reach a high level, eliminating them via the skin would be the most expedient and efficient method.

Medicine and Food

What place do these old, and sometimes outlandish, home remedies have in our current society? It is a fact that modern medicines are easily obtainable these days and they work much faster. However, many of them have the side effect of causing drowsiness. In addition, more and more people have allergies to some of the more common medicines available. More importantly, modern medicines tend to address the symptoms of the underlying problem only and do not remedy the root cause of the illness, which is an imbalance of the body's energies. This leads us to look for alternatives for improving our health and recovering from illness.

There is a principal in Chinese pharmacology that states: medicine and food come from the same source (医食同源). Another says: food remedies are preferred over medical cure (食疗胜于药疗). They demonstrate how closely food and wellness are intertwined in Chinese thought. If you do not want to fall ill, then you must first of all eat wisely. However, if you do become sick, you can also turn to food to help you recover. In essence, you are what you eat.

To have a better understanding of how food remedies work, you must first be familiar with the yin-yang concept, the yin and yang organs, and the various body complexes.

The Yin Yang Concept

Illness, in Chinese principles, is caused by imbalance in the body according to the concept of yin and yang. If there is imbalance, it would soon result in one force engulfing the other. The yin-yang symbol ☯ shows the perfect state of harmony. The circle represents wholeness. The S-shaped curve denotes the dynamic forces of all life, with the bright yin force and the dark yang force pushing against each other to maintain equilibrium. A fragment of each force is embedded inside the opposing force to keep its ferocity in check. To the Chinese, this yin-yang concept is applicable to the universe, the earth, plants, animals, people and even different parts and functions of the human body.

Of course, the concept also applies to food and its ingredients. So, one can eat food with the appropriate properties to restore the body's balance.

Here is a chart to show the yin and yang qualities of common food:

FOOD	HOT	WARM	NEUTRAL	COOL	COLD
BEVERAGE	Hot Chocolate	Hot Coffee	Water	Chilled Cola	Iced tea
FRUIT	Durian	Papaya	Apple	Pear	Watermelon
VEGETABLE	Chili	Chive	Hairy Marrow	Watercress	Angled Luffa
MEAT	Mutton	Beef	Pork	Frog	
POULTRY	Pigeon	Chicken	Quail	Duck	Teal

What is interesting is that the same food product can have different properties depending on what state they are in. Take the longan fruit for instance. When fresh longans are eaten in summer, it has the effect of increasing the yin element, thus cooling ones body. However, eating too much will cause the formation of phlegm, and in extreme situations, giddiness for anaemic people. Dried longans, on the other hand, are no longer cooling, but have acquired yang properties, which is warming and therapeutic. Thus, dried longans are commonly used in soups and tonics and is effective for soothing the heart and brain, and therefore good for relieving insomnia.

To eat for wellness the Chinese way, one must first know how to distinguish a person with yin characteristics from a person with yang characteristics. The table below gives the basic profiles.

BASIC YIN CHARACTERISTICS	BASIC YANG CHARACTERISTICS
Timid	Temperamental
Quiet	Active
Soft voice	Loud and rough voice
Pale looking	Ruddy-faced
Does not perspire easily	Perspires freely
Often feels giddy	Hyperactive
Anaemic	Obese
Limbs feel cold	Gets thirsty easily

A yin person can neutralise her body complex by adding yang foods to her diet. A person with yin characteristics who is anaemic, for example, should eat more liver which is a yang ingredient that builds red blood cells. However, he should not eat too much cooling food as it may result in giddiness.

The yang person can neutralise his body by eating more yin foods. If he feels that the heat in his body is bringing on a sore throat, for example, he can have watercress, a yin ingredient, to bring his body to equilibrium. However, too much heaty food is not recommended for a yang person as it may generate more heat in the body and result in nosebleed, sore throat or constipation.

Yin and Yang Organs

Apart from this, one must also know how the Chinese classify the major organs of the body according to the yin–yang system. The yin organs are the lungs, liver, kidneys, heart and spleen while the yang organs are the large intestines, gall bladder, bladder, small intestines and stomach. These organs are also paired according to yin and yang: lungs with large intestines, liver with gall bladder, kidneys with bladder, heart with small intestines and spleen with stomach. With this understanding, you can better monitor the functions of the various organs which is indirectly linked to the health of the individual.

The lungs filter the air entering the body and help the large intestines with the supply of *chi* to work out the bowels. When waste is effectively excreted, expelling toxins, the hair will be healthy and glossy and the complexion will be clear. In other words, dull and lifeless hair indicates disharmony in the lungs and large intestines. Sorrow and sadness will also affect the health of the lungs.

The liver regulates the flow of blood and *chi* energy to the body and its muscles. It also has a connection to the gall bladder. Healthy, sparkling eyes indicate that the liver is in good order; if not the eyes can be red, dry and irritated with blurred vision. If the white of the eyes are yellow, it could be due to a jaundiced liver. Strong emotions, resulting in stress, can upset the harmony of the liver and gall bladder.

The kidneys receive and filter waste fluid and sends it to the bladder for excretion. It also controls reproduction, growth and development. Hair loss is an indication of weakened kidneys, as is the swelling of hands, legs and the body through water retention. Sometimes, sudden fear can affect the kidneys and bladder.

The heart dominates blood, the blood vessels and the complexion of the face. Its health can be determined by observing the colour and texture of the tongue. When the heart is doing well, the blood in the small intestines are better able to absorb the nutrients from digested food. Excitement and joy will affect the heart and the mind, as mental function is closely related to blood supply. The Chinese believe that one must be calm to maintain the heart's well-being.

The spleen transforms and transports nutrients and water in the body. It regulates blood flow and also affects the quality of the muscles. Appetite and the ability to taste well is related to the health of the spleen, and therefore to the stomach.

Heat

The character for heat (燥) is composed of the ideogram for fire (火) on the left, three objects (品) on the top right, and wood (木) on the bottom right. Together, it shows fire burning the wood and drying things up. Familiar phrases my parents used to describe heat are Summer heat (夏燥), dry heat (干燥) and fiery heat (干火燥).

Excess body heat in hot summer weather can bring about profuse sweating, parched mouth and throat, and constipation.

Dry heat affects the lungs, resulting in dry nose and throat and causing heavy coughing and pains in the chest. This is because of the lack of moisture in the body. Dryness also manifests in dry skin, dry lips and constipation. Urine may be passed in small amounts and is very yellow and cloudy.

The most extreme form of heat is fiery heat. It usually exhibits more intense forms of Summer heat and dry heat. Too much heat can bring about a heaty, hacking cough with yellowish-green phlegm.

Drinking lots of soothing and lubricating brews will alleviate heat. Buddha's Fruit Soup (p 30) and Double-boiled Tatarica Horn with Japonicas Root (p 38) are two classic time-tested recipes. I munched on preserved Buddha's Fruit throughout my trip on the Silk Route. It helped a lot when I was travelling through the desert.

Cold

Cold is obviously associated with the yin element, and eating too much cooling food can introduce excess yin to the body. It injures the yang *chi* of the system in different ways. If cold affects the body superficially, it can result in chills, fever, headache and body pains. If it reaches the meridians, it produces muscle cramps and aches in the bones and joints. If it enters the internal organs, intestinal noises, abdominal pains, diarrhoea and even vomiting may occur.

Like excess heat, excess cold can also bring about a cough. A cooling cough manifests in a running nose, fever and bubbly, clear phlegm. To return warmth to the body, have some Ginger Porridge (page 42).

Dampness

Just as humidity affects clothes, books and leather, the Chinese believe that humidity also affects the body. When there is excess humidity in the body, it will upset the fluid balance and cause water retention. Thus, those with dampness may not only have swollen legs, but also feel lethargic and tired. The blocked flow of energy may cause aches and pains.

Inner dampness can be caused by having too much cold food and drinks. My mother is a great believer in this concept. She never allowed us to eat chilled fruit right out of the fridge. We had to let the fruit stand at room temperature until the condensation evaporated. This way, she said, we would not introduce dampness into our bodies. Grandmother went further and never ate chilled fruit or drank cold drinks. She hardly suffered from rheumatism which is common among old folks.

This is related to why people who have arthritis or rheumatism can tell, by the aches and pains in their bodies, that rain is coming. The humidity or dampness in their bodies will rise before the rain arrives, and the excess humidity blocks the *chi* system, and results in pain.

When a person with a heaty body complex has excess dampness, we call this heat dampness (湿热). This is manifested in a wide variety of skin problems. People with this condition should avoid eating too much crustaceans and shellfish. Mango, coconut and coconut-milk based foods are also unsuitable. If you have loose and messy stools after eating these foods, it is a clear sign that you have heat dampness.

To alleviate heat dampness, try the Similax and Castanea Brew (p 82). Better still, prevent the condition by avoiding the taboo food and drinks mentioned.

Wind

Wind enters the body through the pores of the skin. For those with a heaty body complex, wind is driven out from the body as gas. However, the system of those with a cold body complex cannot easily drive out the wind, thus resulting in its accumulation, especially in the joints.

Windy people may feel the sudden movements of wind as darting pains and aches. Muscle cramps, hay fever and rashes may also manifest. These conditions arise suddenly and subside equally suddenly, but will recur.

Once wind has entered the system, it will travel to all parts of the body.

That is why the Chinese have recorded so many types of wind.

Excess wind and dampness in the body is known as wind dampness (风湿). It causes aches and pains especially in the limbs and lumber region.

If wind dampness is not taken care off in its early stage, wind may penetrate the bones and result in rheumatic pain. Besides drinking brews to drive away the wind, medicated plasters will also help to relieve the aches and pain.

Those with wind in the head (头风) complain of headaches regularly. It could be a person with a heaty body complex where hot wind has moved into the neck and head. Try some Cooling Tea (pg 21) to alleviate the condition. For someone with a cooling body complex suffering from wind, have Grandmother's Ginger Tea (pg 47).

Conclusion

As demonstrated in the examples of the various body complexes, there are a number of common ailments and conditions that affect the body, especially when it is already weak. A sudden change of climate or weather can also bring on ailments as the body is unable to adapt quickly. Think about it: have you felt unwell as you travelled from a warm climate to a cold place or vice versa? Have you fallen ill at the onset of the rainy season?

This is where home brews and food remedies come into their own, building resistance and correcting yin-yang imbalance to restore health.

Food remedies do not always involve herbs. Instead, you can use foodstuff familiar to every household: Grains and beans, nuts and berries, vegetables and tubers, sugar and spices. If herbs are used, most will be common ones which can easily be found in neighbourhood herbal shops.

As you go through the recipes in this book, you will find that many of them are easily prepared through boiling or double-boiling. A few of them can even be eaten as a meal. It is my hope that the information in this book will prove useful and fit easily into your everyday life so that you can maintain good health for the long run.

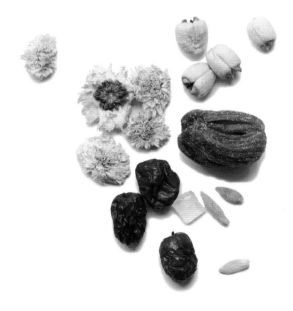

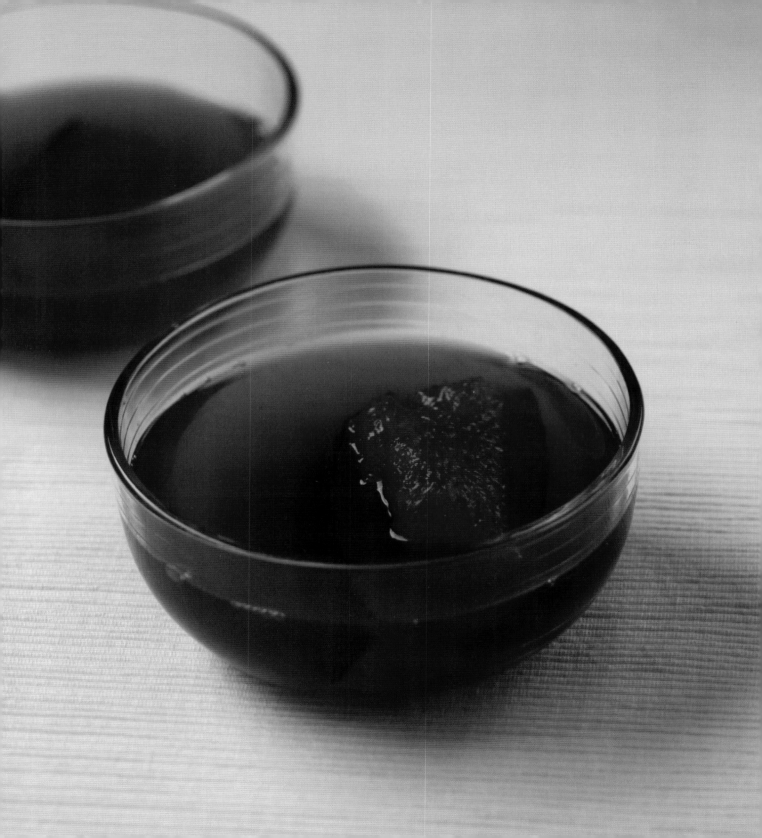

荷叶冬瓜汤

● LOTUS LEAF WINTER MELON SOUP

When Father had fresh winter melon left over from his restaurant, he would ask Mother to prepare this soup for the family. Mother used dried lotus leaves, but, at times, she would use fresh leaves if they were available from her florist.

Father said that this soup is good for clearing fire from the heart (清心火), that is, it cuts down the body heat during hot, dry spells. It is quite a cooling soup!

Do not use too many lotus leaves as it will make the soup taste bitter.

50 g (2 oz) dried lotus leaves
500 g (1.1 lb) winter melon
1½ litres (6 cups) water
100 g (3.5 oz) brown sugar

Rinse and drain the lotus leaves. Cut open the winter melon, remove and discard the pith. Wash the winter melon and cut into big wedges.

Bring 1½ litre (6 cups) of water to a boil. Put in the dried lotus leaves and wedges of winter melon and boil over high heat for 10 minutes. Bring heat to medium-low and simmer the soup for 30 minutes.

Add the brown sugar and continue to simmer for another 30 minutes until the soup has reduced to 1 litre (4 cups).

Cool and serve this sweet soup. The melon wedges can be eaten.

粥
水

● RICE SOUP

Chinese peasants, when cooking rice during the hot season, used to keep a few bowls of rice soup for family members to drink. The Northern Chinese call this cooked rice Porridge Oil or Porridge Water (粥油，粥水), while in the south, it is known as Rice Soup (米汤).

Rice Soup has high nutritional value because it contains the essence of rice grains. All you have to do is to add more water to the pot when cooking rice or porridge and save a few bowls of this soup.

This soup helps to cool the internal organs, cleanse the intestinal tract, prevent constipation, aid digestion and quench thirst during a hot spell. It is best for those who work in the open under the sun and is also good for growing children with heaty body complex.

100 g (½ cup) raw rice
1¼ litres (5 cups) water

Rinse the raw rice briefly and drain. Put the cleaned rice and 1¼ litres (5 cups) of water into a pot and bring to a boil.

Lower the heat to medium and leave to simmer for 5 minutes until the rice grains begin to break up. The rice water should be milky at this stage.

Ladle out 2 cups of Rice Soup. Leave to cool and serve lukewarm.

Do not waste the rice. Continue to cook it until all the water has been absorbed. Lower heat to very low and cook for a further 5 minutes until the rice is thoroughly cooked.

凉茶

● COOLING TEA

I used to accompany my grandmother to her favourite herbal shop and, during the hot season, she would ask the herbalist to pack two portions of this formula for her. Grandmother added brown sugar, saying that it alleviates dampness.

During the long hot spell, you can be sure that every member of our family had to drink this tea to avoid heatiness and rashes. There is no fixed formula for cooling tea and each family has its own, passed down from generation to generation.

In the 1930s, single male Chinese immigrants relied on vendors selling precooked cooling tea to balance their body complex after a hard day's work under the tropical sun. My late father-in-law was a pioneer in selling such herbal teas. Today, to cater to modern needs, tea bags of cooling tea are available. So, you have the choice of brewing a large pot of this tea or use the convenient just-brew-and-drink Chun Chun cooling tea bags.

40 g (1.4 oz) *Shui Oong Fah* (水翁花), *Cleistocalyx operculatus (Roxb.)*
40 g (1.4 oz) *Kong Mui Gun* (岗梅根), *Ilex asprella champ*
20 g (0.7 oz) *For Tan Moh* (火炭母), *Polygonum chinenese Linn.*
10 g (0.3 oz) dried lotus leaf
100 g (3.5 oz) brown sugar
1½ litres (6 cups) water

Rinse the herbs briefly and drain.

Bring 1½ litres (6 cups) of water to a boil, then add the cleaned herbs and bring to a boil again for 5 minutes over high heat. Bring to medium-low heat and simmer for 20 minutes.

Add the brown sugar and continue to simmer the tea for another 20 minutes until it has reduced to 1 litre (4 cups). Ladle out the tea and cool. Discard the herbs. Drink the tea lukewarm.

☯ SALTED LIME BREW

咸酸柑水

Auntie Chan lived along the same row of shophouses as we did in Chinatown. She imported flowers and fruit-bearing plants for the Lunar New Year season. During that time of the year, my nanny would ask her permission to pick up the fallen ripe Chinese lime for pickling. After gathering a large quantity, she would dry the golden limes in the sun until they started to wrinkle. Then she would sprinkle salt on them and preserve them in glass jars.

Whenever one of us children complained about an approaching sore throat, she would prepare this salted lime brew.

This brew is best taken before bedtime or early in the morning before breakfast to prevent the heat from ascending to the upper body (以防上火). In other words, it suppresses latent heat.

So, after the next Chinese New Year, pick the ripened limes from your festive plant and preserve them.

It will take about a week for the limes to dry out suitably. Make a shallow slit on each lime to hasten the process.

4 salted limes
1 teaspoon sugar
250 ml (1 cup) boiling water

Use a spoon or fork and mash up the salted lime in a mug. Add the teaspoon of sugar and mix well.

Pour in 250 ml (1 cup) of boiling water, stir well, and cover the mug. Leave to stand for 10 minutes. Drink lukewarm.

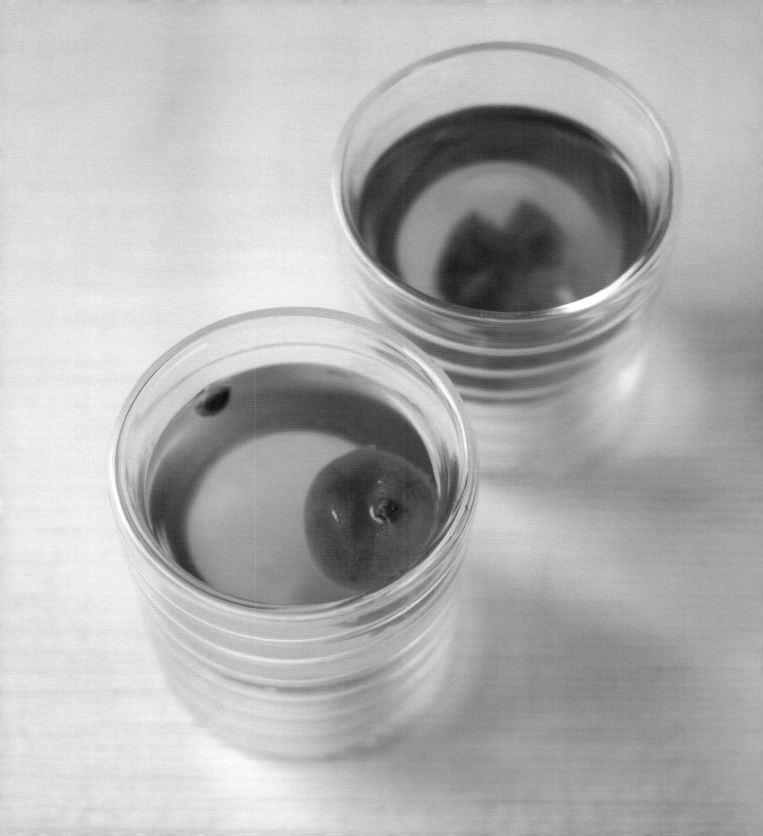

● SWEET FRANGIPANI BREW

This recipe was passed down to me by Ah Sam Por (亚三婆). She and her husband, Ah Sam Goong (亚三公), made a living from selling sweet floral brews. They occupied a small backroom of our neighbour's house, so they had direct access to the backlane where an old frangipani tree grew.

I remember Ah Sam Por picking fallen frangipani flowers every morning and evening. She dried the flowers on a mat until they turned yellowish brown. Then, she would cook this Sweet Frangipani Brew, and she and Ah Sam Goong would sell it and other brews from their pushcart on the streets of Chinatown.

I knew when Ah Sam Por was cooking her Sweet Frangipani Brew because its fragrance would waft over to our house. I once asked her why we drink this brew, and she told me that it alleviates intestinal heatiness (清肠热).

At times, Grandmother bought a small pot of the brew for us to drink. I suggested that we could also pick the flowers and make the brew ourselves. Grandmother frowned and said we must respect other people's trade.

30 g (1 oz) dried frangipani flowers, *Plumeria obtusa L.*,
    available from herbal shops
80 g (2.8 oz) brown sugar
750 ml (3 cups) water

Rinse the dried frangipani briefly and drain. Bring 750 ml (3 cups) of water to a boil, add the frangipani and boil for 5 minutes over high heat.

Bring the heat to medium-low and simmer the brew for 30 minutes. Add the brown sugar and continue to simmer for another 15 minutes until it has reduced to 250 ml (1 cup). Sieve and discard the dregs. Drink the brew lukewarm.

凉粉

● GRASS JELLY

Liang Fen Chao (凉粉草), *also known as Fairy's Grass* (仙草), *is* Mesona chinensis Benth, *and is grown abundantly in Canton province. The plants are harvested in summer and are put through a fermenting and drying process. The dried leaves are then soaked in water and boiled till the liquid becomes black and sticky. This consistency comes from the leaves. The liquid is then put through a sieve and ground rice water is added. It is then left to set into a jelly.*

Grass jelly is very cooling, and is not recommended for very weak people or those with a cooling body complex. However, it is a popular snack during hot spells and is always eaten with a sugar syrup. It can ward off the summer heat, cool the organs and quench thirst.

Grass jelly is available at most markets and found in packets in supermarkets. You can grate the jelly into long strips, add syrup and cold water to make the refreshing drink that is popularly known as Chin Chow.

400 g (14 oz) grass jelly, *liang fen*
1 pandanus leaf
200 g rock sugar
375 ml (1½ cups) water

Chill the grass jelly in the refrigerator till cold. Wash the pandanus leaf and knot it. Rinse the rock sugar briefly.

Bring 375 ml (1½ cups) of water to a boil. Put in the pandanus leaf and rock sugar and boil for 10 minutes over medium heat until 250 ml (1 cup) of syrup remains. Remove the pandanus leaf and leave the syrup to cool, then chill the syrup.

Cut the grass jelly into 2.5 cm (1 inch) cubes. Serve with the syrup.

甜蕃茄

● SUGARED TOMATOES

On one of my visits to northern China, besides the usual sesame seed buns, my host served these sugared tomatoes for my breakfast. She encouraged me to eat more of them, explaining that they would prevent ulcers from forming in the mouth because of the dry heat accumulated in the body during the cold winter months.

I took her advice and ate what she had served. And I was free from those awful mouth ulcers. Since then, I have adopted this snack to prevent mouth ulcers even in the tropics.

2 large ripe tomatoes
2 teaspoons sugar

Wash and pat dry the tomatoes and cut them into round slices. Place the slices of tomatoes on a flat plate and sprinkle sugar evenly on each slice. Leave to stand for 5 minutes before serving.

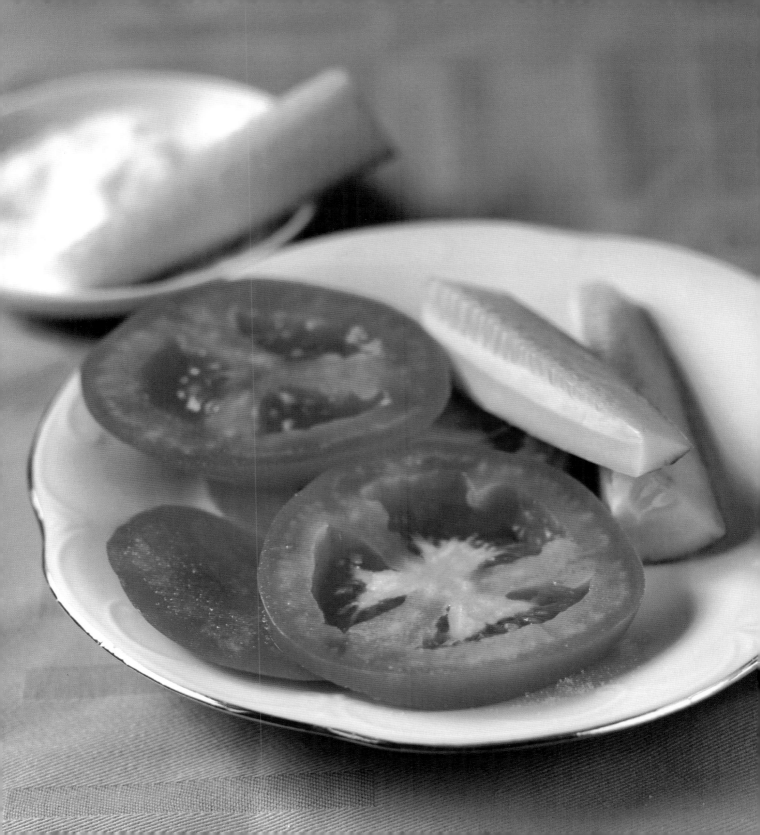

甜青黄瓜

● CUCUMBER WITH SUGAR

From when I was young, I have followed the habit of the workers in Father's restaurant in eating cucumber dipped in castor sugar to prevent sore throat. Eat it once you feel discomfort in your throat before it is too late.

Cucumber is a cooling vegetable, but people with rashes on the body should avoid it as its sap is considered bad for problem skin.

1 medium-sized cucumber
2 teaspoon castor sugar

Wash and pat dry the cucumber. Do not remove skin. Cut off 2.5 cm (1 inch) from both ends of the cucumber and use each tip to rub the cut edges to draw up the cucumber sap. Cut off another 1 cm from each end of the cucumber and quarter the cucumber, if preferred. Wash and pat dry.

Eat the whole cucumber, dipping it in the castor sugar before each bite.

● PIG'S SPLEEN POLYCONATTUM SOUP

As all the members of my family were involved in the restaurant business, we slept late. Thus, the liver latent heat would rise, and one of its effect was bad breath (口臭). Drink this soup over a couple of days and see how your breath improves. Polyconattum *soothes the lungs* (润肺) *while* Prunella *and* Paeonia *alleviates liver heat* (清肝火).

50 g (2 oz) *yok chok, polyconattum*
50 g (2 0z) *har foo choe, Prunella vulgaris L.*
30 g (1 oz) *pak cheuk, Paeonia lactiflora Pall*
2 pig's spleens, *jue wang lei* (猪横脷)
1 piece preserved tangerine peel
2 litres (8 cups) water
2½ teaspoons salt

Trim off the strips of fat from the spleens. Rub the spleens with 2 teaspoons salt. Rinse and drain.

Scald the spleens in hot water for a minute. Rinse and drain. Cut each spleen into 10 cm (4 inch) lengths.

Rinse all the herbs briefly and drain.

Bring 2 litres (8 cups) of water to a boil. Put in all the ingredients and boil over high heat for 10 minutes. Lower heat to medium-low and simmer the soup for 3 hours.

Season with ½ teaspoon salt before serving.

● BUDDHA'S FRUIT SOUP

Ah Mun Sok was a kitchen hand in my father's restaurant. His duty was to clean and prepare raw ingredients for cooking. So, one of Ah Mun Sok's jobs was to clean fresh octopus. He would save the flat, white, surfboard-like internal cartilage of the octopus, and would dry them in the sun until they no longer smelled fishy. He kept them for remedies such as this one.

This recipe is Ah Mun Sok's family heirloom, and he said that Buddha's fruit with dried octopus cartilage alleviates latent heat lumps. These lumps appear on both sides of the neck, just below the jaw line, when children have too much heaty food such as deep-fried snacks. They are usually accompanied by a sore throat and a dry, hacking cough with thick, yellow phlegm. Drink this soup twice and the lumps will disappear.

My research shows that octopus cartilage has medicinal value. No wonder Ah Mun Sok's soup works.

1 Buddha's fruit, *lohan kuo*
4 honey dates, *mut cho*
10 g (0.3 oz) sweet and bitter almond mixture
1 piece dried octopus cartilage, *hoi piew siew* (海漂啸)
300 g (10.5 oz) lean pork
2¼ litres (9 cups) water

Scald the lean pork in hot water for 3 minutes. Rinse and drain.

Wash and dry the Buddha's fruit. Break the fruit into bite-sized bits. Wash and dry the octopus cartilage.

Bring 2¼ litres (9 cups) of water to a boil. Put in all the ingredients and boil for 10 minutes over high heat. Reduce to low and simmer the soup gently for 2 hours. Serve the soup only.

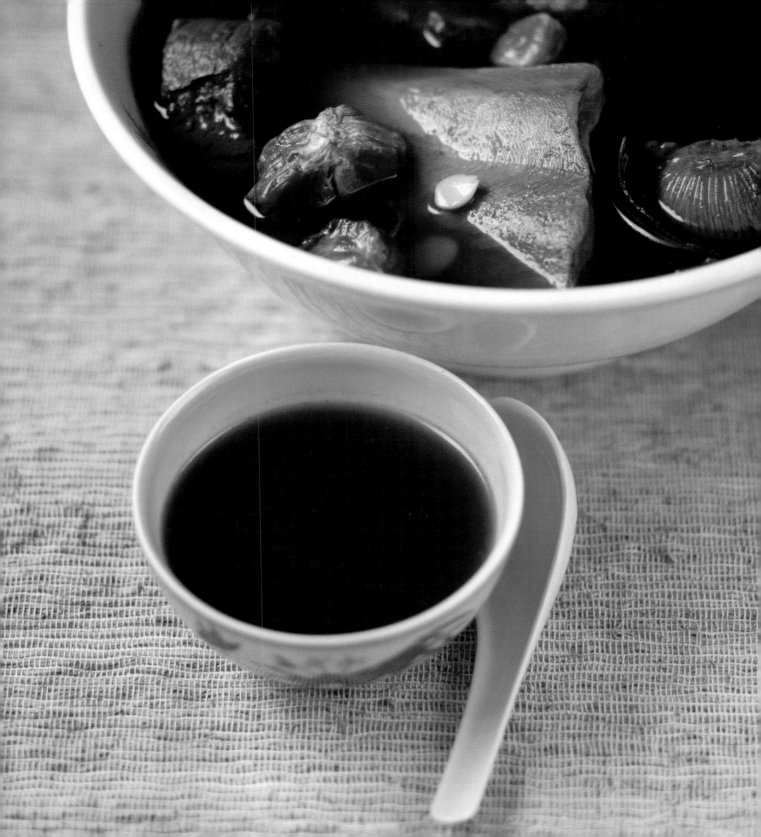

蛋花茶

☯ SUGARED EGG WATER

If you feel your voice getting hoarse from too much yelling or cheering, you should soothe (润) your throat with this brew before things get worse.

Try my nanny's remedy for a hoarse voice (沙哑). This is one of my favourite childhood drinks — it is nice and sweet. Best taken before bedtime; the throat will feel more comfortable the next morning.

30 g (1 oz) rock sugar
2 eggs
250 ml (1 cup) water

Bring 250 ml (1 cup) of water to a boil. Add the rock sugar and lower the heat to medium and simmer for 5 minutes or until the sugar has completely dissolved.

Break the eggs into a bowl and beat lightly for a minute. Remove the sugared water from the heat and stir in the beaten eggs.

Serve lukewarm.

干贝露

☯ SCALLOP ESSENCE

Once, one of my younger brothers had dried, cracked lips and blisters at the corner of his mouth when he returned home from camp during National Service. He could not eat and felt thirsty all the time. He was said to be suffering from acute dry heatiness.

The proprietor of my father's favourite dried seafood shop gave my father this recipe to ease my brother's discomfort. He said that it should be drunk for five consecutive days for mild cases. Should blisters also develop at the tip of the tongue, the essence should be drunk eight days in a row for better effect.

100 g (3.5 oz) dried scallops
375 ml (1½ cups) hot water
¼ teaspoon salt, optional

Wash the dried scallops to get rid of the white powder. Drain. Put the scallops into a double boiler and add 375 ml (1½ cups) hot water. Double boil for 3 hours.

Add salt before serving, if required. Drink the essence lukewarm. The cooked scallops need not be eaten.

Drink this essence for 5 consecutive days to see results.

薏米绿豆粥

● BARLEY AND MUNG BEAN PORRIDGE

Accidents do happen in the kitchen. Whenever any of the cooks or helpers scalded or burnt themselves in my father's restaurant kitchen, Ah Mun Sok would apply first aid. Besides putting on medication, he would quickly cook this porridge for the victim to have. He said that one must quickly clear the heat absorbed during the accident, so that there will be a quick recovery with no complications.

This very cooling dish is also good for those with a very heaty internal complex.

200 g (7 oz) pearl barley
200 g (7 oz) mung beans (green beans)
100 g (3.5 oz) rock sugar
2½ litres (10 cups) water

Rinse the pearl barley and soak in water for 10 minutes. Drain before cooking. Rinse and drain the mung beans and also the rock sugar.

Bring 2½ litres (10 cups) of water to a boil. Put in the soaked barley and mung beans and bring to a boil over high heat. Lower the heat to medium and continue to cook the soup for 1 hour until the barley and mung beans have broken up. Stir and check the water level occasionally and adjust if necessary. The consistency should be a grainy gruel.

Include the rock sugar and continue to cook for a further 5 minutes over low heat. Stir after every minute to avoid the gruel from sticking and burning. Serve the porridge hot.

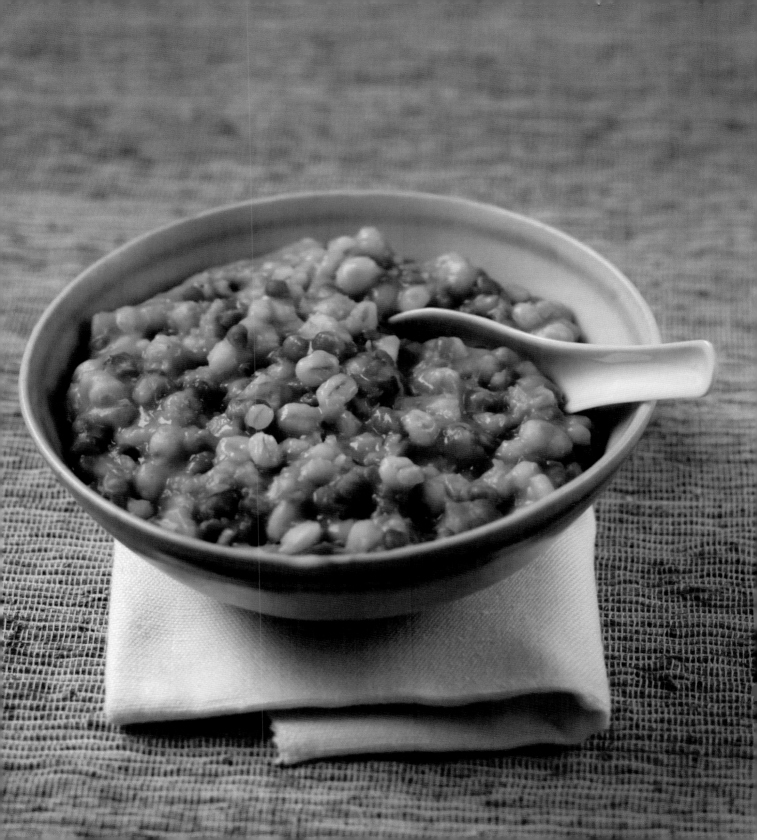

豆腐石膏汤

● BEANCURD GYPSUM SOUP

Gypsum is a limestone found in northern China. It is the coagulant used in making beancurd and has cooling properties.

Drink this soup to quench your thirst, stop heavy perspiration and subside body heat during dry spells. In our family, we also drank this soup when we had blood-shot eyes due to the lack of sleep. I was told that it could prevent conjunctivitis.

200 g (7 oz) soft beancurd, *dao fu*
50 g (2 oz) raw gypsum, *san sek go*, ground finely
500 ml (2 cups) water
½ teaspoon salt

Rinse and cut the beancurd into quarters.

Bring 500 ml (2 cups) of water to a boil. Put in the beancurd and the gypsum and continue to boil for 5 minutes over high heat. Add the salt.

Lower the heat and simmer the soup for 1 hour. Strain the soup and serve with the beancurd.

糖水油条

🌓 FRIED FRITTERS WITH SUGAR WATER

Fried fritters (油条) are also known as yau cha guai (油炸鬼). The elders in my family used to eat porridge with fried fritters. Leftover fritters were never thrown away. Instead, they were eaten the next morning with sugar water to 'open the voice' (开声).

Freshly fried fritters are oily and heaty, but fritters kept overnight are mellow and less heaty because the yeast in the fritters is no longer active.

Thus, these fritters, without the sugar water, are also good for those with excessive stomach acidity.

1 fried fritter, *yau cha guai,* kept overnight
1 teaspoon castor sugar
250 ml (1 cup) hot water

Dissolve 1 teaspoon of castor sugar in 250 ml (1 cup) of hot water. Set aside to cool.

Eat the fried fritter dipped in the sugar water. Drink the sugar water too.

● DOUBLE-BOILED TATARICA HORN WITH JAPONICAS ROOT

Tatarica horn brew is a very common Chinese remedy for bringing down fevers. The Cantonese drink it to alleviate internal heat from the body while the Hokkiens and Teochews drink it more frequently to prevent the accumulation of internal heat.

The horns of saiga antelopes reared in the north-eastern provinces of China are of great medicinal value. They are very cooling and are not recommended for those with cooling body complex, and definitely not for those with asthmatic conditions.

If the high fever does not subside after drinking this brew, a physician should be consulted.

10 g (0.3 oz) *ling yeung kok, Saiga tatarica L.* horn shavings
10 pieces *muk dung, Ophiopogon japonicus (Thunb.) Ker-Gawl*
4 pieces sugared wintermelon
300 ml (1¼ cups) hot water

Rinse the *muk dung* and sugared wintermelon and put them in a mug together with the tatarica horn shavings. Pour in 300 ml (1¼ cups) of hot water, cover the mug and double-boil for 2 hours. Strain and cool the brew before drinking. The wintermelon can be eaten.

Do not discard the remaining cooked ingredients. You may add 250 ml (1 cup) of hot water and 2 pieces of sugared wintermelon and double-boil for 1 hour to make a second brew. Discard the horn shavings and *muk dung* when this second brew is ready.

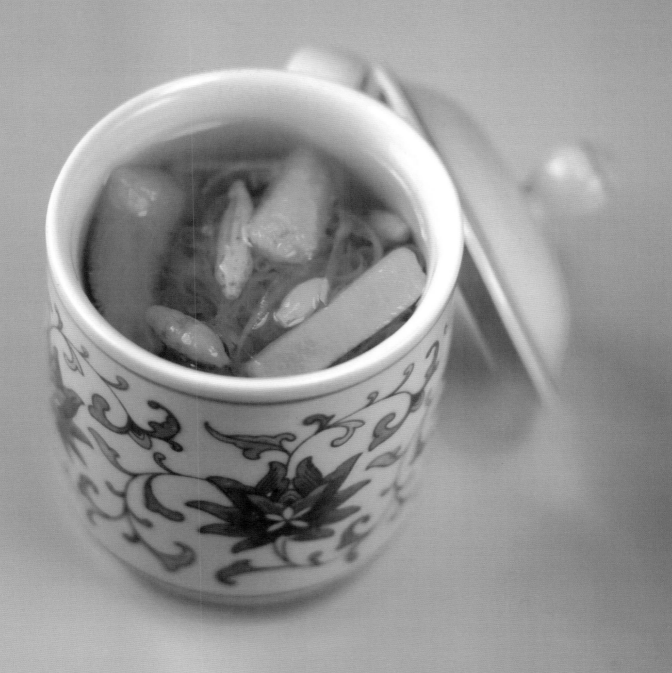

杏仁糊

❀ ALMOND CREAM

My maternal grandmother was an expert in making Almond Cream. She used her granite grinder and slab to grind the almonds and rice grains. There was no such thing as an electric blender then!

Poh-poh made this cream for us when the weather was dry and hot. She said that it prevents dryness of the lungs. In other words, it wards off dry coughs and phlegm. She also said it was good for the complexion.

You can adjust the amount of almonds in this recipe to achieve your favourite aroma and consistency. I enjoy thick, strong Almond Cream.

300 g (10.5 oz) sweet almonds, *nam hung*
50 g (2 oz) bitter almonds, *pak hung*
2 litres (8 cups) water
100 g (3.5 oz) raw rice
100 g (3.5 oz) rock sugar, rinsed

Soak the sweet and bitter almonds together in a little water for 1 hour. Drain. Soak the raw rice grains in 250 ml (1 cup) of water for 1 hour. Reserve the rice water.

Combine the soaked almonds, raw rice, rice water and blend into a thick paste. Strain with a muslin cloth and discard dregs.

Pour the strained almond and rice mixture into a pot. Add 1¾ litres (7 cups) of water and bring to a boil over medium-low heat, stirring all the time. Add the rock sugar. Stir and simmer the mixture until a light, milky consistency is achieved and the almond fragrance is obtained. Check for sweetness and adjust if necessary. Serve the Almond Cream hot.

蒸柿饼

☯ STEAMED PERSIMMONS

Bad eating habits and the accumulation of heatiness in the large intestines are why piles or haemorrhoids develop.

In the old days, when someone in the neighbourhood developed piles, you can be sure that news travelled fast. Gossip was passed and remedies were exchanged!

This simple dish helps to soothe the lungs and large intestines.

3 dried persimmons
30 g (1 oz) rock sugar, rinsed

Remove the stems of the dried persimmons. Wash away the white powder on the dried fruit. Pat dry.

Slice the dried persimmons crosswise into thick slices. Put the pieces on a steaming dish and place the rock sugar on top.

Steam for 30 minutes over medium-low heat until the sugar has dissolved and the persimmons are tender and soft.

Drink the syrup and eat the persimmons.

姜粥

○ **GINGER PORRIDGE**

This porridge is recommended for those who have a bad cold accompanied by a runny nose. Take this porridge to speed up recovery.

The old ginger and fried rice grains will generate heat throughout the body, thus warming up the system and expelling the coolness (驱寒). The runny nose and discomfort will subside soon.

My grandmother used to cook this ginger porridge for herself during the cold, rainy season to keep herself warm.

4 slices old ginger
100 g (3.5 oz) raw rice
750 ml (3 cups) water

Wash the rice grains and drain. Fry the raw rice, without oil, in a wok over very low heat for about 5 minutes until the rice turns golden brown. Cool.

Bring 750 ml (3 cups) of water to a boil. Put in the rice, old ginger and boil for 5 minutes over high heat.

Bring the heat to medium and continue to cook the porridge for 20 minutes till the rice grains have all broken up. Check the water level occasionally and adjust, if necessary.

Serve the ginger porridge hot. The cooked ginger can be eaten.

云吞皮汤

○ **DUMPLING WRAPPER SOUP**

When you catch a chill and have a blocked nose, try this soup. You will perspire after drinking it, indicating that your organs have warmed up to dispel the bad chi (邪气) from your body. Your blocked nose will clear up and you will feel more comfortable.

4 slices old ginger
2 stalks spring onions
50 g (2 oz) leeks
20 dumpling wrappers, *won ton* skins
375 ml (1½ cups) water
½ teaspoon salt
Pinch of pepper

Wash and dry the spring onions and leeks. Cut the spring onions into 5 cm (2 inch) lengths. Smash the white stems lightly with the flat of a cleaver. Slice the leeks diagonally in 2.5 cm (1 inch) lengths.

Bring 375 ml (1½ cups) of water to a boil. Put in the slices of old ginger, the spring onions and the leeks. Bring to a boil again over high heat.

Reduce the heat to medium-low and simmer the soup for 5 minutes. Add the dumpling wrappers, season with salt and pepper and continue to cook for a further 5 minutes. Serve hot. All the ingredients can be eaten.

洋葱面汤

○ **SPRING ONION NOODLE SOUP**

This is a popular dish in northern China where the winters are very cold. It is eaten to warm up the body system.

This noodle soup is also good for those with a weak and cooling body complex. If you are about to catch a chill, this dish will fend it off. Expect to perspire after eating it. You can adjust the degree of hotness by adjusting the seasoning. The northern Chinese love chilli oil as it gives a more fiery effect.

Spring Onion Noodle Soup is unsuitable for those with a heaty body complex or have a dry, hacking cough.

6 stalks spring onions, washed, chopped finely
4 slices old ginger, shredded
100 g (3.5 oz) dried noodles
1 tablespoon oil
500 ml (2 cups) boiling water

1 red chilli, chopped OR 1 tablespoon red chilli oil
2 dashes of pepper
½ teaspoon salt

Heat 1 tablespoon of oil in a saucepan and fry the chopped spring onions and shredded ginger for 2 minutes till fragrant.

Add 500 ml (2 cups) of boiling water, cover the saucepan and bring to a boil. Include the dried noodles and continue to cook over high heat for 5 minutes.

Season with the chilli, pepper and salt. Cook for another 1 minute. Serve immediately.

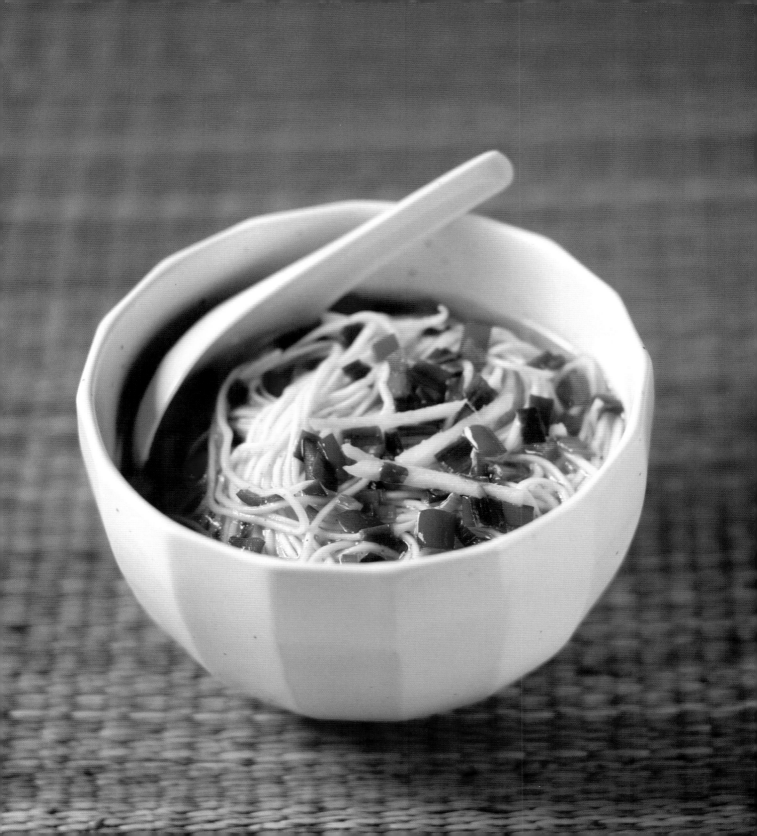

蜂窩茶

● HONEYCOMB BREW

If you have little white sores on the tip of your tongue and inside your mouth, it is an indication that toxic heat (溃热) has developed. It is the combined heat derived from the stomach, heart and liver. When this happens, you will have difficulty chewing and digesting your food.

For mild cases, drinking a glass of lukewarm water with a tablespoon of honey will improve the situation. For more acute ulcers, try this Honeycomb Brew followed by dabbing the sores with honey. By the third day, the sores would have gradually healed.

Do not drink the brew for more than four consecutive days as muk dung should not be taken in large doses. Also, do check your diet and avoid deep-fried and heaty foods.

25 g (0.8 oz) honeycomb, *mut fung wor* (蜜蜂窩)
2 tablespoons honey
20 g (0.7 oz) *muk dung, Ophiopogon japonicus (Thunb.) Ker-Gawl*
1 litre (4 cups water)

Rinse and drain the *muk dung* and also the honeycomb. Bring 1 litre (4 cups) of water to a boil, put in the *muk dung* and honeycomb and boil for 5 minutes over high heat.

Reduce the heat to medium-low and simmer for 1 hour till the liquid is reduced to 250 ml (1 cup). Add the honey and stir well. Strain and cool the brew before drinking.

姜
茶

○ **GINGER TEA**

We have a large number of elderly ladies in our family, so Mother always kept a stock of old ginger root.

Old ginger has the effect of expelling coolness and wind (驱寒驱风) and warming the stomach (暖胃).

Ladies with cooling body complex may occasionally have fainting spells. A bowl of hot ginger tea will help. For additional relief, clean a piece of old ginger root and heat it over a flame. Cut a few slices of the heated root and place them on the forehead, keeping them in place with a folded handkerchief used as a headband.

My grandmother and her friends used this method to 'push the wind from the head' (去头风). They looked like Ninja Turtles!

200 g (7 oz) old ginger
100 g (3.5 oz) brown sugar
375 ml (1½ cups) water

Wash and slice the ginger across the grain slantwise. Leave the skin on.

Bring 375 ml (1½ cups) of water to a boil in a saucepan. Put in the sliced ginger and continue to boil for 5 minutes over medium heat.

Add brown sugar and simmer for another 5-10 minutes till the liquid has been reduced to 250 ml (1 cup). Stir occasionally.

Discard the ginger and serve the tea hot.

大海欖茶

● SWEET STERCULIA TEA

Tai hoi lam literally means 'olive of the big sea'. It is the olive-shaped nut of Sterculia scaphigera Wall found mostly in South China and Southeast Asia.

When the dried nut is soaked in water, its soft shell absorbs water, causing it to swell like a sponge, with a brown, jelly-like substance emerging. For this reason, the nut is also called pung tai hoi (崩大海), meaning 'bursting the big sea'.

Tai hoi lam is considered very cooling and can clear intestinal heat (清肠热). It provides good roughage when constipated (便秘) and is able to restore a hoarse voice due to lack of sleep.

The popular dessert, Cheng Tng, has tai hoi lam as one of its many ingredients.

2 pieces *tai hoi lam* (大海欖) *Sterculia scaphigera Wall.*
30 g (1 oz) rock sugar, rinsed
250 ml (1 cup) water

Soak the *tai hoi lam* in a bowl of warm water for 30 minutes. As the nuts begin to expand, remove the soft skin to help the jelly-like substance of the nuts to fully swell up. Remove the stones and finally, drain away the water. Set aside the brownish jelly.

Meanwhile, bring 250 ml (1 cup) of water to a boil. Add the rock sugar, reduce heat to medium and simmer for 5 minutes or till the sugar has completely dissolved.

Pour the sugared water into a big bowl and add the *tai hoi lam* jelly and stir well. Cover the bowl and leave to stand for 10 minutes before drinking.

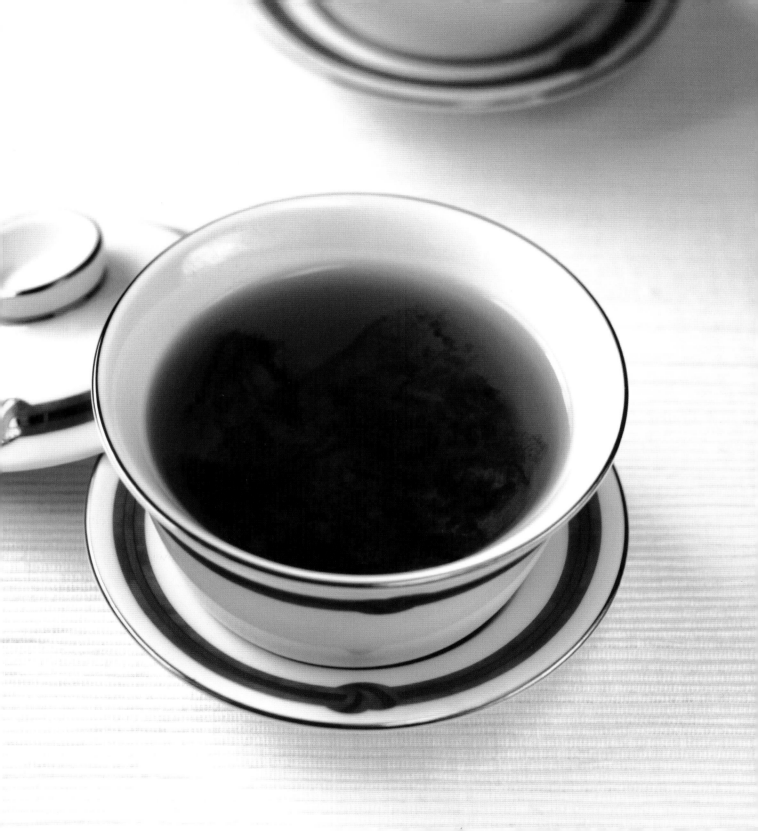

蜜糖红枣茶

☯ HONEY AND RED DATE TEA

This simple tea is my mother's prized rejuvenation recipe. She called it her 'nurture her heart and stabilise the mind' tea.

Red dates soothe the heart (安心) and reinforce the chi system (补气). When the heart is functioning smoothly and the energy system is strengthened, what else can you expect but a good night's sleep.

Red dates are warming, but combined with the cooling honey, this tea is neutral and feeds the yin and yang of the body. Do not forget to remove the stones of the red dates as the stones are heaty.

20 red dates
1 tablespoon honey
750 ml (3 cups) water

Rinse and pat dry the red dates. Remove the stones, but keep the dates whole.

Bring 750 ml (3 cups) of water to a boil. Put in the red dates and boil over high heat for 5 minutes. Reduce heat to medium-low and simmer the tea for 30 minutes or until it has been reduced to 250 ml (1 cup).

Stir in the honey and simmer the tea on low heat for another 5 minutes. Serve warm and eat all the red dates.

安定茶

○ **WELL-BEING TEA**

Do not bring your worries to bed, or else you may have insomnia. An insomniac may, at times, have headaches, feel giddy, experience palpitations, lack concentration, have loss of memory and get fatigued.

If you have insomnia, drink this tea daily for a fortnight. You will soon find yourself sleeping easily and well again. This tea is also beneficial to those who are anaemic.

50 g (2 oz) red dates, stoned
100 g (3.5 oz) black beans
30 g (1 oz) dried longan flesh
1½ litres (6 cups) water

Pan fry the black beans without oil for 5 minutes over medium heat. The skin should split and the white part of the beans should start to turn a light golden brown. Set aside.

Bring 1½ litre (6 cups) of water to a boil. Put in the dates, black beans and dried longan flesh and boil for 10 minutes.

Reduce heat to medium-low and simmer for 1 hour until the liquid has been reduced to 750 ml (3 cups).

Sieve the tea and discard the cooked ingredients. Keep the tea in a flask and drink it through the day.

咸竹蜂茶

● SALTED BAMBOO WASP BREW

These black, round wasps make their hives among the wild bamboo of Szechuan province. When caught during the autumn and winter months, their bellies contain honey. Salt is sprinkled on them for preservation and for alleviating heatiness.

The wasps have soothing and cooling elements which get rid of heaty wind that results in a hoarse voice. So, Chinese opera singers depend on this brew to maintain their voices.

6 salted bamboo wasps, *ham chok foong, Xylocopa dissimilis (Lep.),*
    including a sprinkle of the preserving salt
50 (2 oz) castor sugar
250 ml (1 cup) boiling water

Put the bamboo wasps with the preserving salt into a mug. Mash coarsely. Add the sugar and mix well.

Pour in 250 ml (1 cup) of boiling water and stir. Cover mug and leave to brew for 15 minutes. Strain and drink the brew lukewarm.

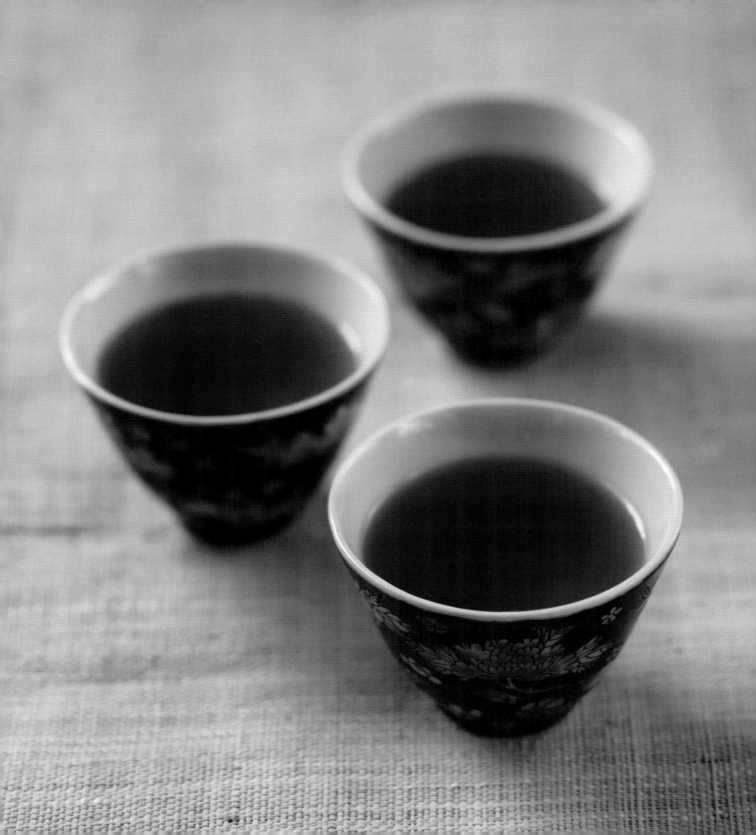

黑
芝
麻
糊

○ BLACK SESAME CREAM

The womenfolk of my family used a granite grinder to prepare black sesame seeds and rice grains for this cream and we children would watch them in fascination.

We were told that Black Sesame Cream benefits our stomachs and intestines. However, the elder ladies ate it for beauty! They said it lubricates their skin and thus improves the complexion. It also prevents hair loss and keeps hair from turning white.

200 g (7 oz) black sesame seeds
200 g (7 oz) raw rice
100 g (3.5 oz) rock sugar, rinsed
2 litres (8 cups) water

Soak the raw rice in 500 ml (2 cups) of water for 2 hours. Retain the water. Rinse and drain the black sesame seeds. Pan fry the sesame seeds in a wok without oil over low heat for 3 minutes till fragrant. Dish out and leave to cool.

Combine the fried black sesame seeds, soaked rice and rice water. Grind or use a blender to grind the mixture into a thick paste. Sieve through a muslin cloth into a saucepan and discard the dregs.

Add 1½ litres (6 cups) of water into the saucepan and bring to a boil over medium-low heat, stirring all the time.

Add the rock sugar and stir, simmering the mixture until it becomes a thin creamy paste. Check for sweetness and adjust, if necessary. Serve hot.

鮮
鴨
肾
汤

● DUCK GIZZARD SOUP

This remedy will help if thyroiditis is detected early. If you have an enlarged thyroid, fast palpitation and your hands shake when you stretch your arms out in front of you, have this soup.

For mild cases, drink it daily for a week and the heart palpitation will slow down. For severe situations, you may want to drink this soup every day for two weeks. Place an order for fresh duck gizzards with your poultry vendor to ensure a ready supply.

6 fresh duck gizzards
1 tsp salt
500 ml (2 cups) water

Peel off the thick brownish-yellow layer from each duck gizzard. Clean and rub the duck gizzards thoroughly with 1 teaspoon of salt. Rinse well. Score the gizzards in a criss-cross fashion. Keep them whole.

Use a cast-iron wok and pan fry the gizzards without oil over low heat for about 5 minutes until the gizzards are dry.

Pour in 500 ml (2 cups) water, cover the wok and bring to a boil over high heat for 10 minutes. Continue to cook over medium heat for another 10 minutes until the soup has reduced to 250 ml (1 cup).

Discard the gizzards and serve the soup lukewarm.

菊
花
茶

● CHRYSANTHEMUM TEA

If your eyes are tired, bloodshot and have a thick discharge, it is time for you to drink this chrysanthemum tea to alleviate heat rising to the upper part of your body (以防上火).

In my family, besides drinking this tea, we also used part of it, including the brewed flowers, to clean the eyes. Do this for a couple of days and your eyes will be refreshed and bright again.

Also, refrain from eating deep-fried, spicy and oily food so as to avoid adding more heat to the unbalanced body.

30 g (1 oz) dried chrysanthemum flowers,
750 ml (3 cups) boiling water
2 teaspoons sugar, optional

Warm a teapot with boiling water. Discard the water and put in the chrysanthemum flowers and sugar, if desired.

Pour in 750 ml (3 cups) of boiling water. Cover the teapot and brew the tea for 15 minutes. Serve the tea warm.

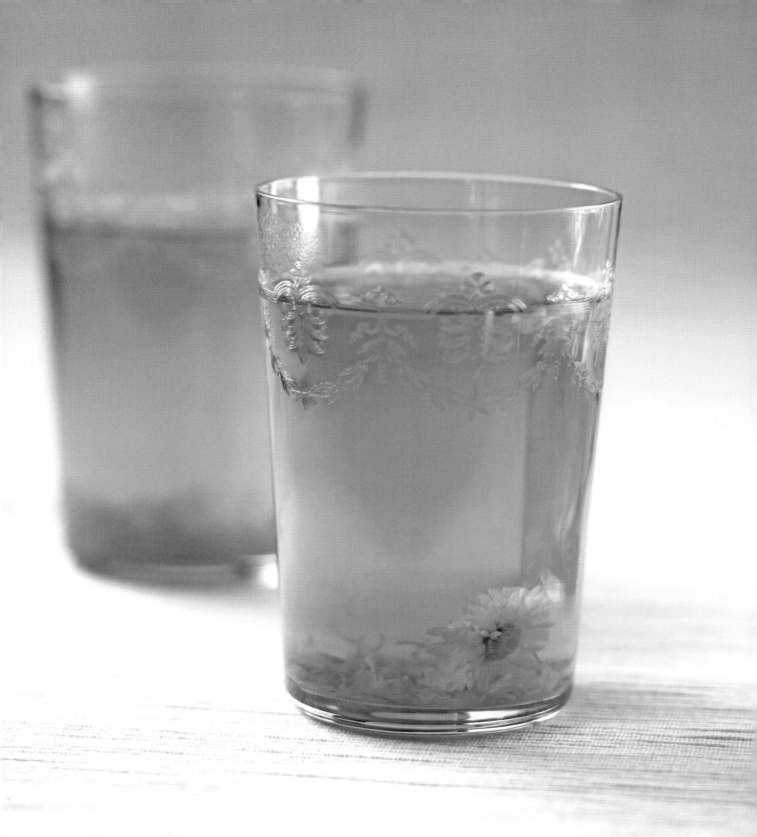

七菜汤

● SEVEN VEGETABLE SOUP

I got this fabulous recipe from one of my herbal masters who swore that "it could lower hypertension". The elders in my family were so excited about it, although no one in the family had hypertension!

Have this soup consecutively for seven days, preferably eating the potato to comfort the stomach in case this soup proves too cooling. After that, have it once a week.

Just look at the colourful line up of ingredients: Yellow potato to benefit the stomach and spleen, orange carrot for the liver, white water chestnut for the lungs and large intestines, pale yellow Spanish onions for the stomach, red tomato for the heart, green celery for the liver and black or purple laver for the kidneys.

No wonder this soup cleanses all the major organs of the body. When the body is well-tuned, one's blood pressure will, of course, be normal.

1 potato, skinned and wedged
1 carrot, skinned and wedged
6 water chestnuts, skinned and sliced thickly
½ Spanish onion, skinned and wedged
1 tomato, wedged
2 stalks Chinese celery, cut into 5 cm (2 inch) lengths
1 piece laver, from Japanese supermarkets
1¾ litres (7 cups) water

Bring 1¾ litres (7 cups) of water to a boil. Put in potato, carrot and water chestnuts and boil for 5 minutes. Reduce heat to medium-low and simmer for 15 minutes, then add onion, tomato and celery. Continue to simmer for another 30 minutes until it has reduced to 1 litre (4 cups).

Finally, add the laver and remove from heat. Do not season this soup. The cooked vegetables may be eaten, if you wish.

● CATFISH AND BLACK BEAN SOUP

The catfish has whisker-like barbels, thus its name. For the same reason, the Cantonese call it Old Man Fish (老人鱼) and Old Uncle Fish (伯父鱼). It is also called tong sut yu (塘虱鱼). The character (塘) means 'pond' and (虱) means 'bug'. The name refers to the catfish's habit of burying themselves in the mud of rivers and ponds like bugs.

Although there is a belief that fish without scales are considered poisonous, the scaleless catfish is the poor man's ingredient for building blood. Thus, this soup is effective in increasing blood formation and chi circulation. No wonder my father used to cook it for the anaemic womenfolk.

Remember to chop off the small bit of red flesh on the catfish's head, if any, since it is said that this bit can cause dizziness.

1 large or 2 medium catfish, *tong sut yu*, about 500 g
200 g (7 oz) black beans, *hak dao*
10 black dates, *hak cho*
20 g (0.7 oz) old ginger
3 litres (12 cups) water

Pan fry the black beans without oil for 5 minutes. Rinse and dry the black dates. Smash the ginger with the flat of a cleaver. Gut and clean the fish. Scald the fish in hot water for 2 minutes. The pale, silvery coating of the fish will come off. Rinse and drain.

Bring 3 litres (12 cups) of water to a boil. Put in the black beans and cook over high heat for 15 minutes. Lower heat to medium-high and continue to cook for 30 minutes. Include the black dates, ginger and catfish. Simmer for 2 hours on medium heat till reduced to 1 litre (4 cups). Adjust liquid if necessary. Serve with cooked ingredients.

淮山蔗汁

● SUGARCANE JUICE WITH DIOSCOREA

The old ladies in the neighbourhood used to make this brew to ward off dry coughs. My mother followed this recipe and I also use it.

First, I had to differentiate the types of coughs. A runny nose with white, bubbly phlegm was from a cooling cough. A blocked nose with thick, yellow phlegm indicated a dry, hacking and heaty cough, with heat locked in the lungs.

This remedy is for the latter type of cough, effective for soothing the lungs and restoring the general health of the stomach. It also expels the phlegm and stops the cough once the lungs have been lubricated.

Children will enjoy drinking the sweet sugarcane juice and munching on the dioscorea.

150 g (5 oz) dried *wai san, dioscorea*
750 ml (3 cups) water
750 ml (3 cups) fresh sugarcane juice

Soak the *wai san* for 1 hour, drain. Boil the soaked *wai san* in 750 ml (3 cups) water over low heat for 1 hour until the *wai san* is almost transparent. The liquid should have reduced to 250 ml (1 cup).

Put half of the cooked *wai san* and all the water into a double-boiler. Add the 750 ml (3 cups) of fresh sugarcane juice and double-boil for 1½ hours over medium-low heat.

Serve the dioscorea and sugarcane juice together.

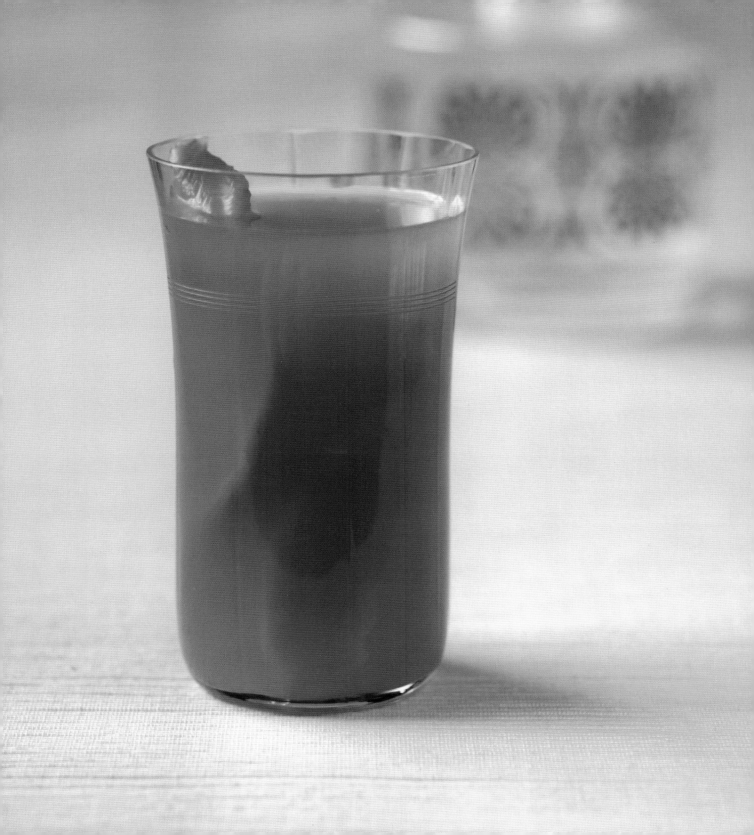

鲤鱼赤小豆汤

⑤ CARP AND GRAM BEAN SOUP

Swollen limbs in old folks indicate cold and dampness in their kidneys due to weakened chi *circulation. When our elders had this soup to alleviate dampness and water retention, they gave some to us children to drink. They said it could also cleanse our urinary tract to aid unobstructed urination.*

My grandmother said that in China, carp were reared in ponds where they ate the nuts of the ferox plant. Ferox nuts also alleviate dampness, as will gram beans.

1 carp, *lei yu*, about 600 g (1.2 lb)
200 g (7 oz) gram beans, *chaik siew dao*
20 g (0.7 oz) old ginger
10 g (0.3 oz) preserved tangerine peel
2 litres (8 cups) water
1 teaspoon oil

Remove the gills of the carp. Do not scale or gut. Rinse thoroughly and drain. Rinse and drain the gram beans. Pan fry without oil for 5 minutes. Cool. Smash the ginger with the flat of a cleaver. Rinse the tangerine peel briefly.

Bring 2 litres (8 cups) of water to a boil. Put in the fried gram beans, cover and boil for 15 minutes. Bring heat to medium-low and simmer for 30 minutes or till the beans are soft.

Meanwhile, heat a wok with 1 teaspoon of oil. Fry the ginger till fragrant. Put in the carp and fry till light golden on both sides. Transfer the fish and ginger into the soup. Add the tangerine peel and simmer for 1 hour on medium-low or till it has reduced to 1 litre (4 cups). Check and adjust liquid if necessary. Do not season the soup. Serve hot without the carp and beans.

青白欖咸話梅茶

○ OLIVE AND SALTED PRUNE BREW

This brew is a remedy for many things. It can be used to give relief to a sore or inflamed throat, it can quench thirst, and also alleviate bloatedness caused by eating too much food that is not easy to digest.

Chewing fresh Chinese green olives will help relieve a sore throat. Swallow the juice but spit out the pulp as it may cause indigestion.

Fresh Chinese green olives are available from Chinese tidbit shops only during the Chinese New Year season, so be sure to put them on your shopping list with your new year goodies.

6 fresh or dried Chinese green olives, *lam*
6 dried salted plums
1 teaspoon castor sugar, optional
750 ml (3 cups) water

Wash the olives and break them open by pounding them lightly with a pestle. Keep stones intact.

Bring 750 ml (3 cups) of water to a boil in a saucepan. Put in the olives and salted prunes and boil for 5 minutes over high heat.

Reduce the heat to medium and simmer for 20 minutes till the liquid has been reduced to 250 ml (1 cup). Add the sugar, if desired.

Strain the brew and serve warm.

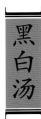

○ BLACK AND WHITE SOUP

The name of this soup comes from the black fermented beans and the white of the spring onion stems. This is a very common remedy for cough and colds accompanied by muscle and bone ache.

Drink the soup very hot and eat up the cooked vegetables. Go to bed quickly and cover yourself up with a blanket. You will perspire in a short while. This is called 'baked perspiration' (焗汗). Change your wet clothes. After perspiring, you will feel more comfortable and the body fatigue and aches will ease.

10 g (0.35 oz) light fermented black beans, *tam dao si,*
8 stalks spring onions
4 slices old ginger, shredded
¼ teaspoon salt
375 ml (1½ cups) water

Rinse and dry light fermented black beans. Mash coarsely.

Use only the white stems of the spring onions. Cut the stems into 5 cm (2 inch) lengths. Smash lightly with the flat of a cleaver.

Bring 375 ml (1½ cups) of water to a boil. Put in the light fermented black beans and boil for 5 minutes. Include the spring onions and ginger, then continue to boil for 3 minutes. Season with salt and stir well.

Serve the soup very hot. The cooked vegetables can be eaten.

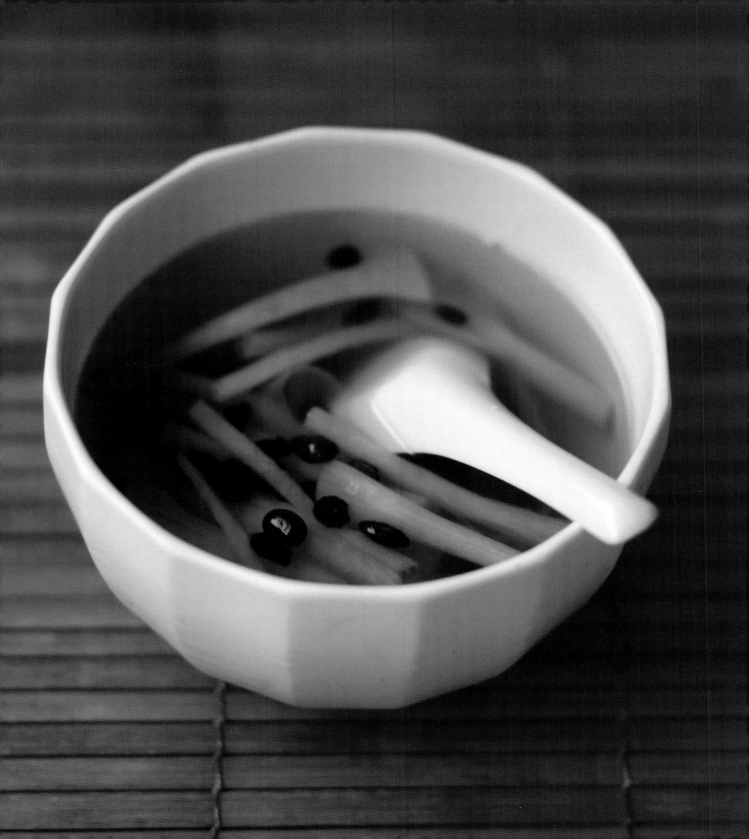

炒
白
果

○PAN-FRIED GINKGO NUTS

Children may urinate frequently at night because of weak bladders. So, the nannies of the neighbourhood served delicious and fragrant pan-fried ginkgo nuts to their charges before bedtime to strengthen the bladders.

In olden China, the lady-in-waiting of a bride would give her pan-fried ginkgo nuts as they set off on the sedan chair journey to the groom's home village. This was to ensure that there was no need to make any convenience stops along the way! So, for those who are planning a long journey where you think toilet facilities may be lacking, do eat a few-pan fried ginkgo nuts before you start your journey.

Pan-fried ginkgo nuts should not be eaten over a long period; just once or twice will be sufficient.

10 ginkgo nuts

Shell the ginkgo nuts. Remove the brownish membrane, then rinse, drain and pat dry the nuts.

Slit open the top of the nuts and remove the tiny sprouts as they are bitter.

Heat a wok and pan-fry the nuts without oil for 10 minutes, stirring all the time until the nuts have dried up. Remove and cool before serving.

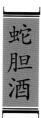

● SNAKE GALL BLADDER WINE

When my father prepared snake broth (蛇羹) in the restaurant, he would save the gall bladders for Grandmother to make this wine for dispelling rheumatism.

You can place orders for snake gall bladder from the game vendor in the Chinatown wet market. Do not worry if the snake is poisonous or not. Just tell the vendor that it is for making snake gall bladder wine. In fact, some believe that the more poisonous the snake, the more effective the gall bladder!

2 snake gall bladder, *sei tam*
750 ml (3 cups) Chinese rice wine

Put 750 ml (3 cups) of Chinese rice wine in a bottle and include the snake gall bladder.

Break the gall bladders with a stirrer and seal the bottle.

Leave the wine to stand for 1 month before using. Drink 2 tablespoons at bedtime.

☯ LOTUS SEED AND PAK HUP PORRIDGE

Sometimes, a recipe has more than one remedial purpose. Take this porridge, for instance. My grandmother ate it to reinforce her memory (增强记憶). Mother said it is good to overcome insomnia (克服失眠). We children were given it to aid digestion and improve our appetite (帮助消化 增进食欲). My nanny insisted that it helps to settle her mind, strengthen her spleen and warm up her stomach (宵神健脾暖胃).

So, we had a big pot of this porridge for the whole family. This dish is not an instant remedy, but should be eaten regularly to be effective.

50 g (2 oz) lotus seeds, *leen chee*
50 g (2 oz) *pak hup, lilium brownii*
100 g (3.5 oz) raw rice, rinsed
2¾ litres (11 cups) water
½ teaspoon salt

Bring 1½ litres (6 cups) of water to a boil. Put in the lotus seeds and continue to boil for 45 minutes over medium heat. Drain and rinse the lotus seeds under cold, running water. Rub skins off and soak the lotus seeds in cold water. Drain before use.

Rinse and drain *pak hup*. Bring another 1¼ litres (5 cups) of water to a boil. Put in the rice and boil for 10 minutes, then add the lotus seeds. Continue to boil the porridge over medium heat for 15 minutes.

Include the *pak hup* and cook for a further 25 minutes over low heat or till the rice grains have broken up. The lotus seeds and *pak hup* should be tender, but remain whole. Check the water level and add more water, if necessary. Add salt to taste and serve hot.

莲子百合粥

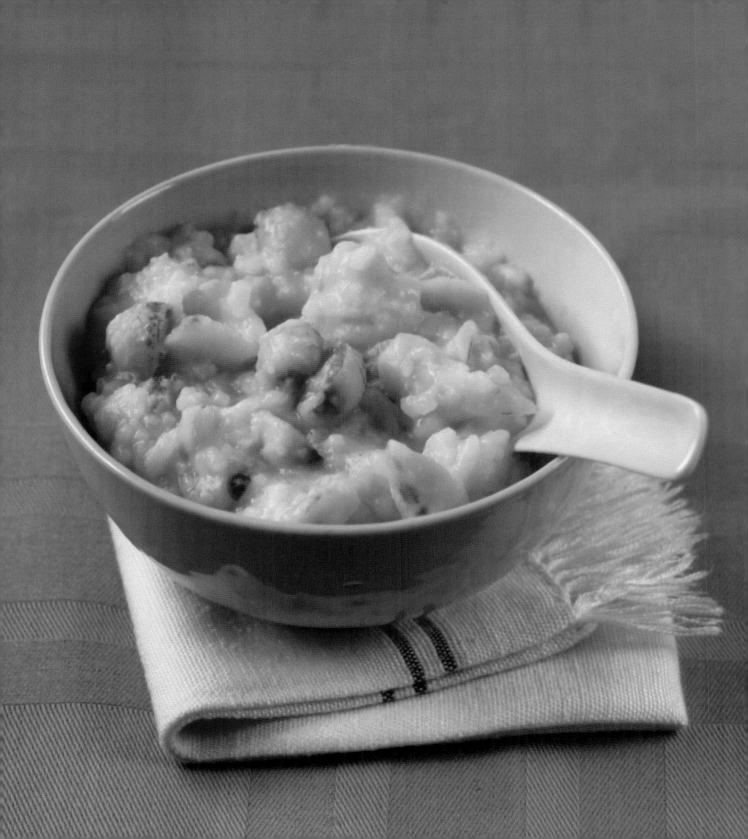

杞子茶

☯ MEDLAR SEED TEA

My grandmother had very good eyesight, and so did my mother. Some nights, the last thing they did before going to bed and the first thing they did in the morning was to prepare this tea. They said it was good for strengthening eyesight.

You have to start before your eyesight weakens, and this tea has to be taken over a long period, say on alternate days for two or three months.

If your eyesight is already fading, have this tea for a longer period. It is possible to do this without adverse side effects because medlar seeds are a neutral ingredient.

20 medlar seeds, *kei chee*
125 ml (½ cup) boiling water

Rinse and drain the medlar seeds. Put the medlar seeds in a cup with a cover.

Pour in enough warm water to just cover the medlar seeds. Cover and leave to soak overnight.

The next morning, pour in 125 ml (½ cup) of boiling water into the cup of soaked medlar seeds. Cover and leave to brew for 5 minutes. Serve. The seeds should be eaten.

冬菇茶

⑤ MUSHROOM TEA

I remember that it was Dr Tong, our family physician, who gave my father this recipe. The womenfolk were told that the brew works for their beauty while it would lower the blood pressure of the men. So, this tea has the effect of alleviating hypertension and lowering cholesterol.

Drink this tea on alternate days for a couple of weeks to see effects.

4 dried Chinese mushrooms
750 ml (3 cups) water

Soak the mushrooms in 1 cup of water for 5 minutes. Drain and squeeze out excess water. Discard the mushroom water.

Bring 500 ml (2 cups) of water to a boil. Put in the mushrooms and boil for 15 minutes over medium heat or till it has reduced to 250 ml (1 cup).

Remove the mushrooms and squeeze dry. Keep the cooked mushrooms for other recipes. Serve the tea hot or warm.

黑
芝
麻
炖
何
首
乌

○ DOUBLE-BOILED BLACK SESAME & POLYGONUM TONIC

Polygonum is traditionally used by the Chinese to promote hair growth. Used together with black sesame seeds and dried longan flesh, it makes a tonic for the hair.

My younger aunts would sprinkle fried black sesame seeds into their cups of longan tea, while the older aunts would have this double-boiled tonic. I followed both their tea and tonic and it really works. You should see the long, black tresses of the elder ladies on hair-washing day.

20 g (0.7 oz) *hoi sau woo, polygonum*
20 g (0.7 oz) black sesame seeds
20 g (0.7 oz) dried longan flesh
500 ml (2 cups) hot water

Rinse and drain the *hoi sau woo*. Pan fry the black sesame seeds without oil for 3 minutes until fragrant.

Put the *hoi sau woo* and dried longan flesh into a double-boiler. Add 500 ml (2 cups) of hot water and double-boil for 1 hour.

Add the pan-fried black sesame seeds and continue to double-boil the tonic for another 1 hour.

Strain the tonic and drink it lukewarm before bedtime.

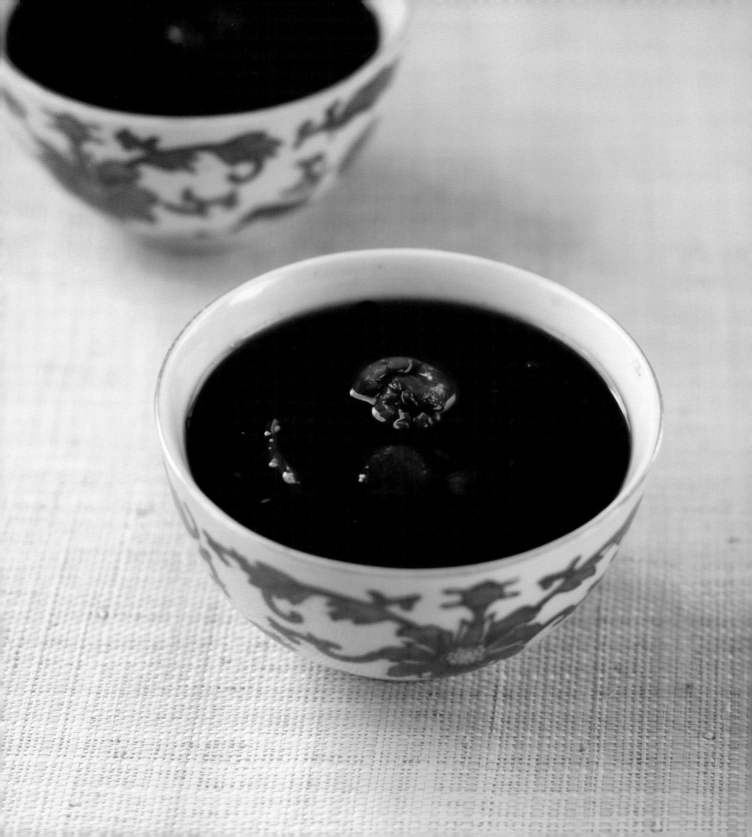

发
菜
粥

● FATT CHOY PORRIDGE

After feasting during the festive season, the stomach may be upset and bloated. This porridge, my grandmother's speciality for 'flushing away bloatedness'' (清除胃胀), will help adjust and cleanse the digestive system.

Fatt choy is very high in fibre, so expect to move bowels after having this porridge.

30 g (1 oz) *fatt choy, nostoc flagelliforme*
100 g (3.5 oz) raw rice
½ teaspoon salt
1½ litres (6 cups) water

Soak the *fatt choy* in water for 15 minutes. Drain. Rinse and drain the rice.

Bring 1½ litres (6 cups) of water to a boil. Put the rice into the pot, cover, and bring to a boil again. Lower heat to medium and cook for 45 minutes.

Include the cleaned *fatt choy* and continue to cook for 15 minutes or till the rice grains are broken up. Check and add more liquid, if necessary.

Season with salt to taste before serving.

止
咳
汤

☯ COUGH RELIEF SOUP

If you have a recurring dry heaty cough, drink this soup to stop your cough completely.

The olives and dried oysters alleviate heat while the honey dates and mango stones soothe the lungs. Save the mango stones after eating the fruit. Wash and then dry them in the sun.

Expect thick yellow phlegm after drinking this soup, but it should go away after a while.

6 fresh or dried Chinese green olives, *lam*
50 g (2 oz) honey dates, *mut cho*
50 g (2 oz) dried oysters, rinsed
2 dried mango stones, *mong guo wat*, available from herbal stores
1½ litres (6 cups) water

Wash and dry the olives. Lightly break open the olives with a pestle, keeping the stones intact.

Bring 1½ litres (6 cups) of water to a boil. Put in all the ingredients and continue to boil for 10 minutes. Reduce heat to medium and simmer for 1 hour or till the soup has reduced to 500 ml (2 cups).

Strain and discard the ingredients. Serve the soup warm.

茅根竹蔗水

● IMPERATA AND BAMBOO SUGARCANE BREW

Chinese mothers traditionally made this brew for their children during the first few days of measles or chicken pox to help reduce the itch and cleanse the body of toxic elements.

During the hot season, this brew is good for quenching the thirst. Mao gun is a very cooling root, so please use it sparingly.

20 g (0.7 oz) *mao gun, Imperata cylindrica Rhizoma*
4 sticks bamboo sugarcane, *chok cheh*, about 15 cm (6 inch) each
10 water chestnuts
300 g (10.5 oz) carrot
2½ litres (10 cups) water

Wash and scrub the bamboo sugarcane. Cut each stick into 3 thin slices lengthwise with a cleaver. Do not remove skin.

Scrub the mud off the water chestnuts and lightly break open each one with the flat of a cleaver. Do not skin.

Skin and cut the carrot into wedges. Rinse and drain the *mao gun*.

Bring 2½ litres (10 cups) of water in a big pot to a boil. Put in all the ingredients and bring to a boil again. Allow to boil for 10 minutes, then lower heat to medium–low and simmer for 1½ hours.

Serve the brew while it is still warm. The cooked ingredients, except the *mao gun*, can be eaten.

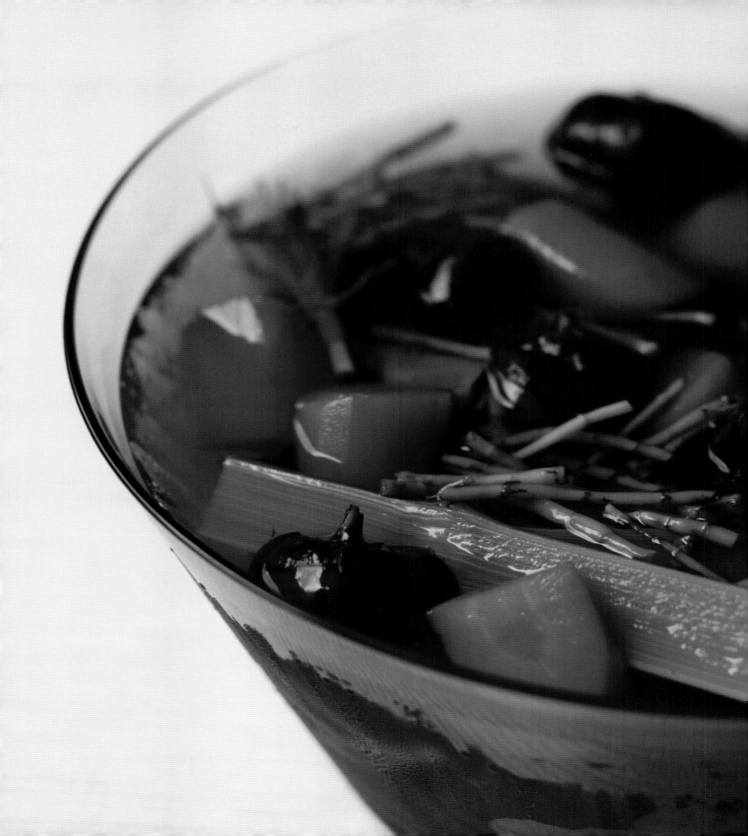

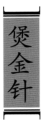

● MUMPS RELIEF BREW

My grandmother picked through the egg seller's stock to find duck's eggs with greenish-blue shells. Duck's eggs with white shells have no remedial effect.

This brew is effective in reducing the swelling of mumps and alleviating heatiness in the body. It is not an old wives' tale — Chinese physicians practise it. Take this brew twice daily and repeat for three days.

Traditionally, a smooth paste of deep purple indigo powder and water is applied on the swollen parts of the face to ease the discomfort caused by the swelling.

1 duck's egg with greenish-blue shell
10 dried lily buds, *kum chum*
50 g (2 oz) rock sugar, rinsed
750 ml (3 cups) water

Wash and dry the ducks egg. Soak the dried lily buds in water for 5 minutes. Squeeze them dry and make a knot at the centre of each stalk.

Boil 750 ml (3 cups) of water in a pot. Put in the ducks egg and dried lily buds and bring to a boil again. Reduce the heat to low and allow to simmer for 30 minutes.

Add the rock sugar and continue to simmer for another 30 minutes until the brew has reduced to 250 ml (1 cup).

Discard the egg and dried lily buds. Cool the brew before serving.

猪横脷淮山汤

● PIG'S SPLEEN DIOSCOREA SOUP

One of my overweight aunts developed diabetes around the age of 40. She had herself to blame as she had a very sweet tooth. She was given this recipe by a friend and was asked to drink the soup for three months, twice a week.

I could see that she was not as tired as before and her doctor confirmed that her diabetes was under control. My aunt insisted that this soup was her life saver so I quickly recorded it in my food remedies notebook.

50 (2 oz) dried *wai san, dioscorea*
50 g (2 oz) *pak kei, astragalus*
50 g (2 oz) gram beans, *chaik siew dao*
40 g (1.5 oz) corn silk, *suk mai so*
2 pig's spleens, *jue wang lei*
2½ teaspoon salt
2 litres (8 cups) water

Soak the *wai san* for 1 hour, then drain. Trim the fat from the spleens. Rub the spleens with 2 teaspoons salt. Rinse and drain. Scald the spleens in hot water for 1 minute. Rinse and drain. Cut each spleen into 10 cm (4 inch) strips.

Rinse all the other herbs briefly and drain. Bring 2 litres (8 cups) of water to a boil. Add the *wai san* and continue to boil for 30 minutes at medium heat. Reduce heat to low and simmer for another 30 minutes. Add all the remaining ingredients and continue to simmer for 1½ hours.

Season with ½ teaspoon salt before serving. Serve warm. The cooked herbs, gram beans and pig's spleen can be eaten.

● OYSTERS, SEAWEED AND KELP SOUP

This is another time-tested remedy for those with a thyroid problem due to a lack of iodine. For those with hypertension, substitute the oysters with lean pork. Drink this soup once a week, one cup twice each day, for a few months to see results.

100 g (3.5 oz) raw oysters
30 g (1 oz) dried seaweed, *hoi tai*
30 g (1 oz) dried kelp, *kuan po*
1¼ litres (5 cups) water
½ teaspoon salt, optional

Rinse and drain oysters. Rinse and drain the dried seaweed and dried kelp.

Bring 1¼ litres (5 cups) of water to a boil. Put in all the ingredients and boil again over high heat for 10 minutes.

Reduce the heat to medium-low and simmer the soup for 45 minutes or until it has reduced to 500 ml (2 cups). Season with salt if desired.

Sieve the soup, discard the cooked ingredients, and serve.

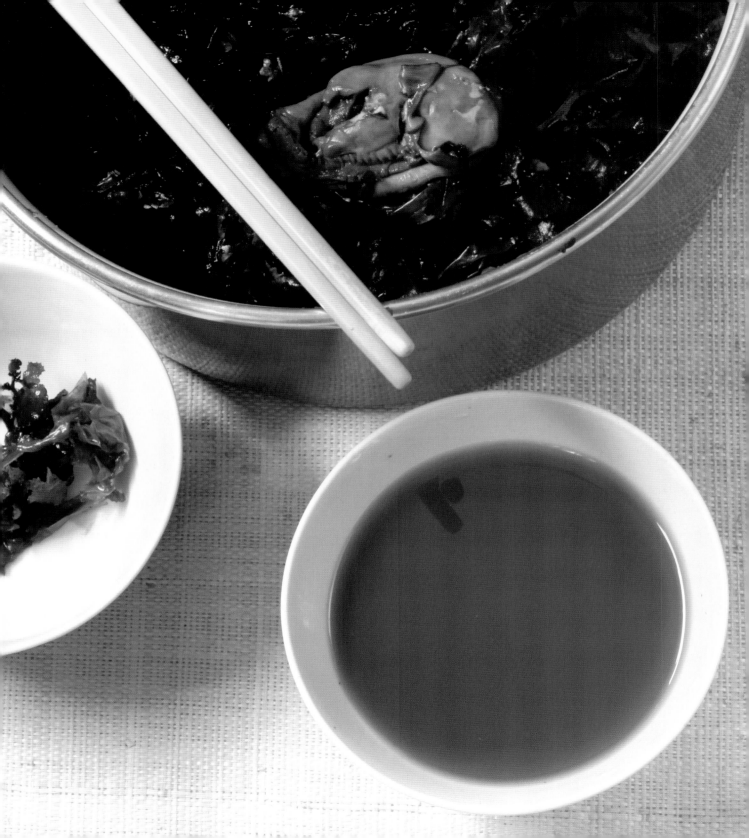

土茯苓栗子壳清汤

☯ SMILAX AND CASTANEA BREW

Hong Kong is a very congested city. People leave home early in the morning for work and return only late at night. Their feet are crammed in socks and shoes all day, and itchiness and rashes develop. This type of problem feet is known as Hong Kong Feet (香港脚). You can get Hong Kong Feet in New York or Singapore!

A friend used this remedy to fight Hong Kong Feet. Drink the soup three to five times a week. Boil ten extra pieces of Castanea *in water and soak your feet in the warm water. The itchiness will stop and the sores will be under control.*

Smilax has the efficacy of releasing dampness and accumulated toxic elements. Castanea, *the shell of the Chinese chestnut, alleviates heat and toxic elements.*

150 g (5 oz) *toh fook ling, Smilax glabra Roxb.*
4 pieces *lut zi hog, Castanea mollissima Bl.*
6 crystallised Chinese figs, *mo fa kuo*
500 g (1.1 lb) sugarcane
2½ litres (10 cups) water

Rinse and cut figs into halves. Wash and scrub the sugarcane. Cut into 15 cm (6 inch) lengths, then split into 3 thin slices lengthwise with a cleaver. Do not remove skin. Rinse and drain the *toh fook ling* and *lut zi hog*.

Bring 2½ litres (10 cups) of water to a boil in a big pot. Put in all the ingredients, making sure to separate the pieces of *toh fook ling*. Boil for 10 minutes then reduce heat to medium-low and simmer for 2 hours or until the brew has reduced to 500 ml (2 cups). Serve lukewarm.

For a second brew, add 1½ litres (6 cups) of hot water and simmer on medium-low heat for 1 hour till reduced to 500 ml (2 cups).

蚌肉绵茵陈汤

● CLAM AND ARTEMISIA SOUP

When one of my uncles developed jaundice, one of the neighbours quickly recommended this remedy. She said this is what they had for jaundice in China. I was given the job of picking out the clam meat every two days.

My research confirms that min yan chan is a cooling herb which helps to relieve jaundice caused by liver problems. Clam meat also benefits the liver.

Sure enough, my uncle's jaundice decreased, and together with appropriate medication, he recovered quickly.

1–1½ kg (2.2 – 3.3 lb) fresh clams, depending on size
40 g (1.5 oz) *min yan chan, Artemisia capillaris Thunb.*
150 g (5 oz) lean pork
1½ litres (6 cups) water
½ teaspoon salt

Scald the fresh clams with boiling water for 1 minute, stirring them around. The shells should partially open. Discard clams that are firmly and fully closed. Pick out the clam meat, rinse and drain.

Wash and drain the *min yan chan*. Scald the lean pork with boiling water for 3 minutes and drain.

Bring 1½ litres (6 cups) of water to a boil. Add the *min yan chan* and clam meat and continue to boil over high heat for 10 minutes.

Reduce the heat to medium-low and simmer the soup for 1 hour or until it has reduced to 500 ml (2 cups).

Season the soup with salt to taste, then sieve. Serve the soup lukewarm.

淡菜皮旦粥

☯ DRIED MUSSELS & CENTURY EGG PORRIDGE

What happens when you have a family member with a cooling body complex and is unable to consume too much cooling food, yet he has latent heat?

Serve this porridge as it combats latent heat and neutralises the body complex (清内热及平行体内状况). This is because dried mussels and century egg have a light cooling effect.

50 g (2 oz) dried mussels
1 century egg
100 g (3.5 oz) raw rice
2 litres (8 cups) water
1 teaspoon salt

Clean the mussels and rinse. Soak them in 250 ml (1 cup) of warm water for 1 hour. Drain, but retain the water. Remove the coating of the century egg to expose the shell. Shell the egg, rinse and pat dry. Cut the egg into quarters and set aside.

Add enough water to the water in which the mussels were soaked to make 2 litres (8 cups). Bring to a boil.

Rinse the raw rice. Put it in the boiling water and cover. Bring to a boil again and then lower the heat to medium-low and cook for 20 minutes or until the rice grains begin to break up. Add the dried mussels and continue to cook for 40 minutes, checking the water level and adding more, if necessary.

Include the century egg and continue to cook for another 10 minutes. Season the porridge with salt before serving.

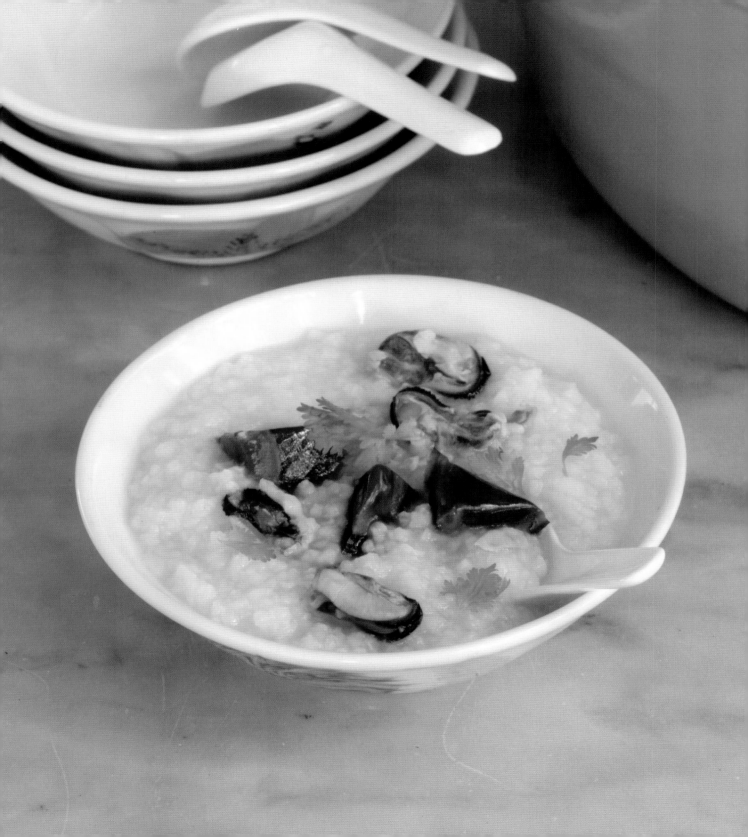

烫鸡蛋

☯ EGG FOR BRUISES

This remedy is for external use only and is a handy one to get rid of bruises.

Grandmother said that for severe bruises, you can slit open the hard-boiled egg and insert a silver coin in the yolk before rubbing. The silver object will draw out the toxic elements and become black.

Rub the bruise for five minutes with the warm egg then rub the area with Teet Dar Chaow (跌打酒). The bruise will become purplish-blue and slightly swollen the day after the application. This is the clotted blood dissipating. Repeat the whole process once or twice a day and the bruise will heal quickly.

Remember, do not eat the egg! Soak the blackened silver coin in vinegar and polish it till it shines again.

1 medium-sized chicken egg
500 ml (2 cups) water
Cotton handkerchief

Bring 500 ml (2 cups) of water to a boil in a small saucepan. Put in the egg, cover the saucepan and bring to a boil.

Reduce the heat to medium low and cook the egg for 20 minutes.

Transfer the egg into a bowl of tap water and allow to stand for 5 minutes. Remove the egg, pat dry and shell it.

Quickly wrap the egg in a cotton handkerchief and use it to rub over the bruise until the egg has cooled off.

Discard the egg after use. Do not eat it.

止
咳
葱
头
包

○ **SHALLOT RICE WRAP**

The children of our family grew up with this Shallot Rice Wrap. Whenever we had a bad cold, coughing up white bubbly phlegm, our nannies would rub our chests and backs with this wrap.

This was to warm up our lungs and dispel the wind from the chest. Used with other remedies for a cold, we were ensured a good night's sleep with less coughing. What a relief!

8 shallots
200 g (7 oz) hot cooked rice
Cotton handkerchief

Skin the shallots, wash and pat dry. Smash them with the flat of a cleaver, but keep whole.

Spread open the handkerchief and place the hot, cooked rice in the middle. Make a well in the rice and put the smashed shallots in the cavity. Cover the shallots with rice.

Bring the four corners of the handkerchief together and twist it into a bundle.

Use the wrap to gently rub the chest and back to expel wind. Discard the rice and shallots when the bundle has cooled down.

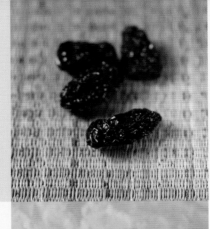

Black dates
Hak cho
Hei zao
黑枣
Pheonix dactylifer

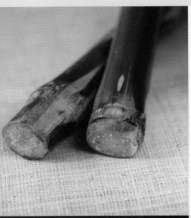

Bamboo sugarcane
Chok cheh
Zhu zhe
竹蔗
Saccharum sinense Roxb.

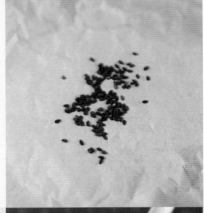

Black sesame seeds,
Hak sze ma
Hei zi ma
黑芝麻
Sesamum indicuma

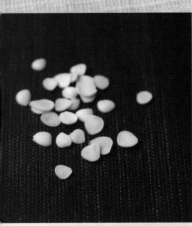

Sweet almonds (bigger nuts)
Nam hung
Nan xing
南杏
Prunus L.

Bitter almonds (smaller nuts)
Pak hung
Bei xing
北杏
Prunus armeniaca L. var. ansu Maxim

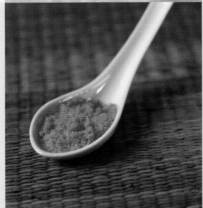

Brown sugar
Wong tong
Huang tang
黄糖

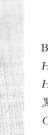
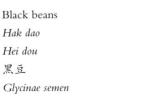

Black beans
Hak dao
Hei dou
黑豆
Glycinae semen

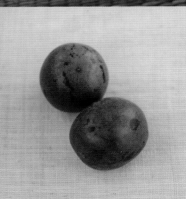

Buddha's fruit
Lor hon kuo
Luo han guo
罗汉果
Momordica grosvenori Swin

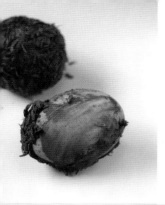

Century egg
Pei tan
Pi dan
皮蛋

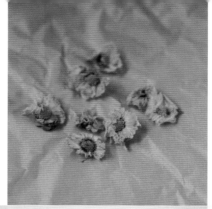

Dried chrysanthemum
Kok far
Ju hua
菊花
Chrysanthemum morifolium
Chrysanthemum indicum

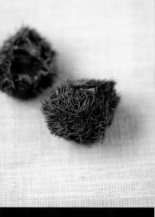

Chestnut shells
Lut chee hog
Li zi ke
粟子壳
Castanea mollissima Bl.

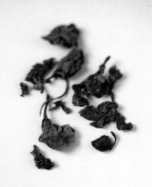

Dried frangipani
Gai dan far
Ji dan hua
鸡蛋花
Pulmeria rubra

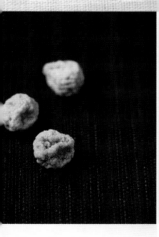

Chinese figs
Mo fa kuo
Wu hua guo
无花果
Ficus carica

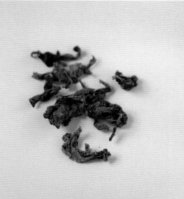

Dried kelp
Kuan po
Kun bu
昆布
Giner primus

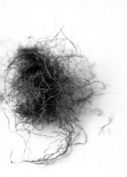

Corn silk
Suk mai so
Su mi xu
粟米须
Zea mays

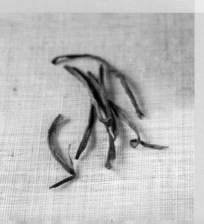

Dried lily buds
Kum chum
Jin zhen
金针
Hemerocallis

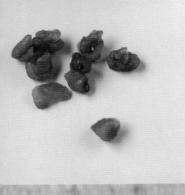

Dried whole longan flesh
Guai yuen
Gui yuan
桂圓 龙眼肉
Dimocarpus longana Lour.

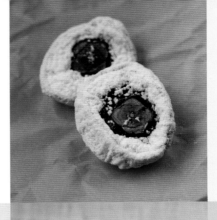

Dried persimmons
Chi paing
Shi bing
柿饼
Diospyros kaki

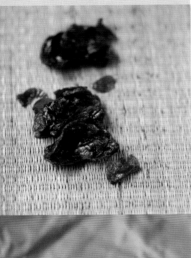

Dried peeled longan flesh
Guai yuen
Gui yuan
桂圓 龙眼肉
Dimocarpus longana Lour.

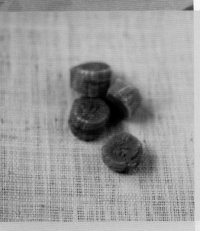

Dried scallops
Kong yu chee
Gan bei
干贝
Pectinidae

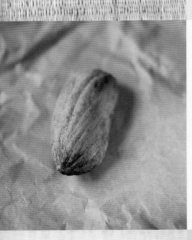

Dried mango stones
Mong guo wat
Mang guo ke
芒果核
Mangifera

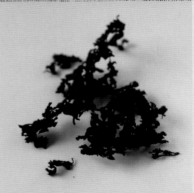

Dried seaweed
Hoi doi
Hai dai
海带
Porphyra

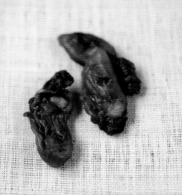

Dried oysters
Hou see
Hao shi
壕豉
Ostreidae

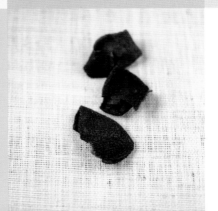

Dried tangerine peel
Chan pei
Chen pi
陈皮
Citrus reticulata Blanco

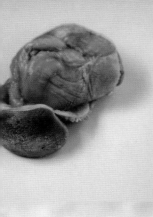

Duck's gizzard
Nyarp shun
Ya shen
鸭肾

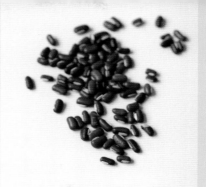

Gram beans
Chaik siew dao
Chi xiao dou
赤小豆
Vigna angularis

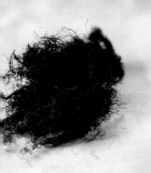

Hair moss
Fatt choy
Fa cai
发菜
Nostoc flagelliforme

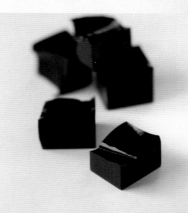

Grass jelly
Leung cho
Liang chao
凉草
Mesona chinensis

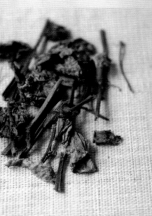

For tan moh
Huo tan mu
火炭母
Polygonum chinense Linn.

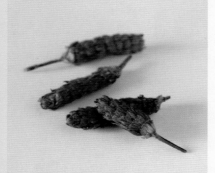

Har foo choe
Xia gu chao
夏枯草
Prunella vulgaris L.

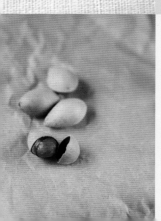

Ginkgo nut
Pak guo
Bai guo
白果　银杏
Ginkgo biloba

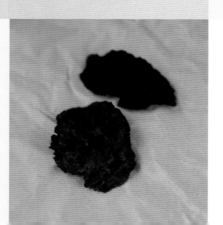

Hoi sau woo
He shou wu
何首乌
Polygonum multiflorum Thunb

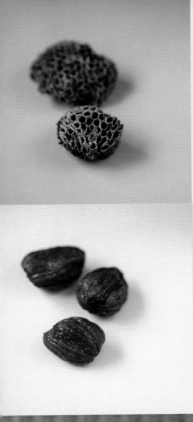

Honeycomb
Mut fung wor
Mi feng wo
蜜蜂窝

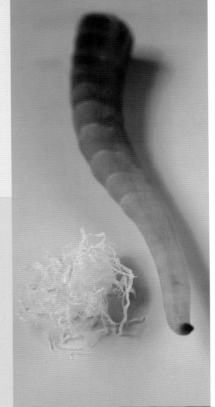

Tatarica horn
Ling yeung kok
Ling yang jiao
羚羊角
Saiga tatarica L. horn

Honey dates
Mut cho
Mi zao
蜜枣
Ziziphus zizyphus

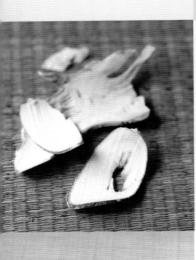

Kong mui gun
Gang mei gen
岗梅根
Ilex asprella Champ.

Lotus seeds
Leen chee
Lian zi
莲子
Nelumbo nucifera Gaertn.

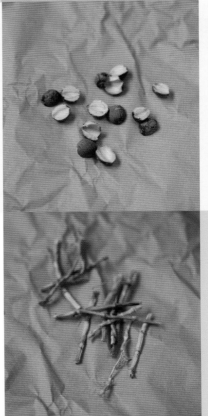

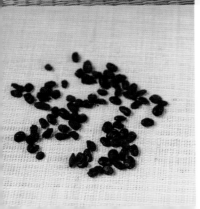

Light fermented black beans
Tam dao si
Dou shi
豆豉
Glycinae semen

Mao gun
Mao gen
茅根
Imperata cylindrica Rhizo

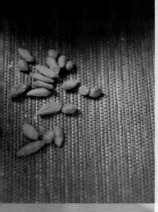

Medlar seeds / Wolfberry
Gei chee
Qi zi
枸子
Lycium chinense Mill.

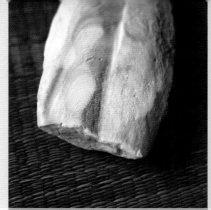

Octopus cartilage
Hoi piew siew
Hai piao xiao
海漂啸

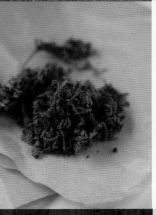

Min yan chan
Mian yin chen
绵茵陈
Artemisia capillaris Thunb.

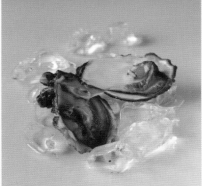

Oysters
Hou
Hao
蚝
Ostreidae

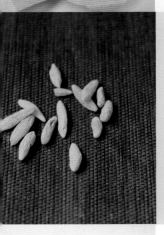

Muk dung
Mai dong
麦冬
Ophiopogon japonicus
(Thunb.) Ker-Gawl.

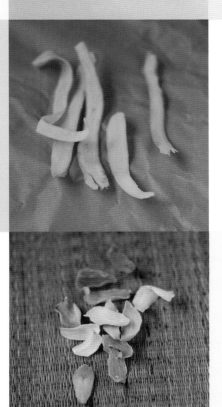

Pak cheuk
Bai shao
白芍
Paeonia lactiflora Pall.

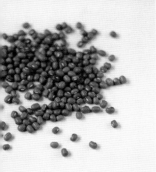

Mung beans
Lok dao
Lu dou
绿豆
Vigna radiata

Lily bulb
Pak hup
Bai he
百合
Lilium brownii

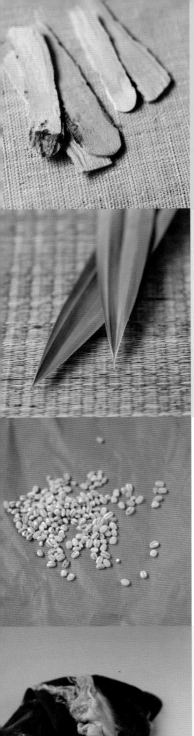

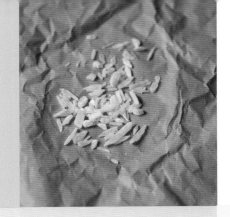

Pak kei
Bei qi
北芪　黄芪
Astragalus membranaceus Bge.

Raw gypsum
San sek go
Sheng shi gao
生石膏

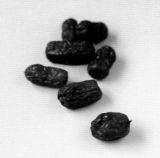

Pandanus leaf
Heung lan yip
Xiang lan ye
香兰叶
Pandanus utilis

Red date
Hung cho
Hong zao
红枣
Ziziphus jujuba Mill.

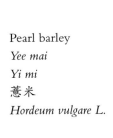

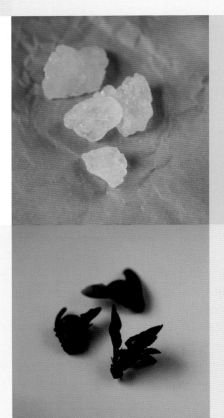

Pearl barley
Yee mai
Yi mi
薏米
Hordeum vulgare L.

Rock sugar
Peng tong
Bing tang
冰糖

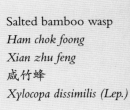

Pig's spleen
Jue wang lei
Zhu heng li
猪横脷

Salted bamboo wasp
Ham chok foong
Xian zhu feng
咸竹蜂
Xylocopa dissimilis (Lep.)

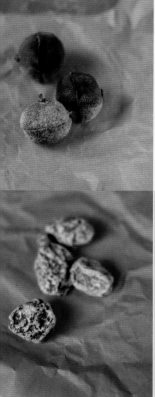

Salted limes
Shuen gum
Suan gan
酸柑
Calamondin

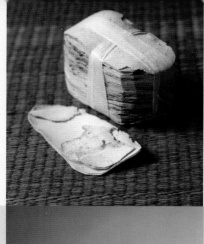

Toh fook ling
Tu fu ling
土茯苓
Smilax glabra Roxb.

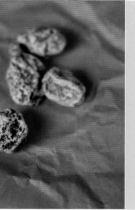

Salted plums
Wah mui
Hua mei
话梅
Prunus

Wai san
Huai shan
淮山
Dioscorea batatas Decne.

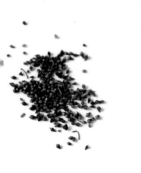

Shui oong fa
Shui weng hua
水翁花
Cleistocalyx operculatus (Roxb.)

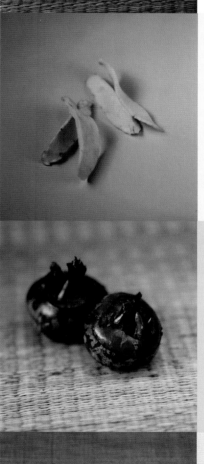

Water chestnuts
Ma tai
Ma ti
马蹄
Eleocharis dulcis

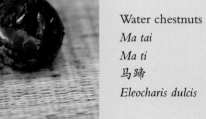

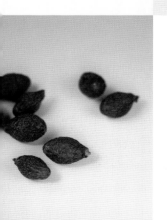

Tai hoi lam
Ta hai lan
大海榄
Sterculia scaphigera Wall.

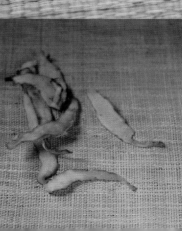

Yok chok
Yu zhu
玉竹
Polyconattum officinale All.

INDEX